A History of Caesarean Birth

From Maternal Death to Maternal Choice

A History of Caesarean Birth

From Maternal Death to Maternal Choice

Thomas F. Baskett
MB BCh BAO (The Queen's University of Belfast)
FRCS (C), FRCS (Ed), FRCOG, FACOG, DHMSA

Professor Emeritus, Department of Obstetrics and Gynaecology
Dalhousie University, Halifax, Nova Scotia, Canada

Clinical Press 2017

On Caesarean delivery

" *A child …..if it cannot be delivered using easier or more common methods, and it becomes apparent that the mother will otherwise die undelivered .*"
    François Rousset, 1581

" *I would never advise such a procedure where there is so much risk without any hope at all.*"
    Ambroise Paré, 1579

" *When the fetus is extraordinarily strong, the passage narrow, the pubic bone flat, it is more than necessary to perform this operation because there is no other way out.*"
    Scipione Mercurio, 1596

" *But I do not know that there ever was any law, Christian or Civil, which doth ordain the martyring and killing the mother, to save the child.*"
    François Mauriceau, 1683

" *This detestable, barbarous, illegal piece of inhumanity.*"
    Fielding Ould, 1742

" *With respect to the child, it is the gentlest and most certain of all the methods we can employ for terminating labour.*"
    Jean-Louis Baudelocque, 1790

" *Employed with discernment, and when the female can support its formidable dangers, it may be perfectly successful, and then becomes a brilliant triumph of art over powerless nature.*"
    Jacques-Pierre Maygrier, 1836

" *The caesarean operation should not be regarded per se as a very dangerous procedure, and should not be held in the dread with which it was long contemplated.*"
    Robert Harris, 1894

" *Normal women come to us demanding a cesarean delivery to avoid the agonies of childbirth. While none would grant them this request, it is well to remember that what is fantasy today may be a fact tomorrow.*"
    Paul Humpstone, 1920

© Clinical Press Limited 2017

All rights reserved. No part of this publication may be reproduced, stored in a retrieval system, or transmitted in any form or by any means , electronic, mechanical, photocopying, recording or otherwise, without prior permission of the copyright owner

While the advice and information in this book is believed to be true and accurate at the time of going to press, neither the author, the editors, nor the publisher can accept legal responsibility for any errors of omissions that may be made. The publisher makes no warranty, express or implied, with respect to the material conatined herein

Published by: Clinical Press Ltd., Redland Green Farm, Redland, Bristol, BS6 7HF, UK.

British Library Cataloguing in Publication Data

Baskett, Thomas F.
A History of Caesarean Birth
From Maternal Death to Maternal Choice

1. Caesarean Birth, History,

New and revised illustrations in this book by Mark Goddard

ISBN 978-1-85457-065-9

Cover illustration: 'Operation césarienne'
(From J.P. Maygrier, Midwifery Illustrated, 1836.)

Contents

	Page number
Foreword	vii
Preface	ix
Acknowledgements	x

Chapter

1.	Caesarean birth in folklore, legend and myth	1
2.	The lexicon of caesarean birth	6
3.	Post mortem caesarean delivery	11
4.	Self–performed caesarean section	23
5.	Traumatic caesarean delivery	29
6.	Caesarean delivery by lay persons	34
7.	Religion and caesarean birth	40
8.	Development of medically performed caesarean section	47
9.	Evolution of the surgical technique of caesarean section	82
10.	Extraperitoneal caesarean section and peritoneal exclusion techniques	97
11.	Lower uterine segment caesarean section	107
12.	Caesarean hysterectomy	119
13.	Anaesthesia for caesarean delivery	128
14.	Modern era of caesarean birth	138
15.	Caesarean birth by maternal choice	159
16.	Some caesarean 'firsts'	169

Foreword

It is a great pleasure to write a foreword for this excellent book on the History of Caesarean Birth. Professor Thomas Baskett in not only an Obstetrician and Gynaecologist par excellence with his clinical, research and teaching track record, but is a well-known medical historian. The sub text of the title is aptly labeled 'From maternal death to maternal choice'. This highlights that caesarean section was introduced to avoid maternal deaths due to ruptured uteri or infection following prolonged and obstructed labour; and now women request caesarean birth as the procedure has been made safe by asepsis, antisepsis, antibiotics, better anaesthesia, blood transfusion and good surgical techniques. Professor Baskett explores the history of various aspects of this common surgical procedure in sixteen chapters of his book. The first chapter is justifiably devoted to folklore, legend and myth surrounding caesarean birth. The second chapter explores the lexicon of caesarean birth – why the name Caesarean was used, as it is well known Julius Caesar was not born by abdominal surgery. The research in this area is new and worth reading. The historical aspects of postmortem caesarean section are explored in chapter 3. It is of interest to note that such a procedure existed from ancient times for cultural or religious reasons. The chapter concludes with postmortem caesarean in recent times to save the mother's or baby's lives, or both.

The sad tales of self-performed caesarean section and cases of traumatic caesarean birth are dramatically represented, with liberal quotations from the original papers. Caesarean section by lay persons is virtually unknown today but some of the earliest caesarean deliveries were by the medically unqualified, and there is a vivid description of one such procedure in Uganda more than 130 years ago. Religion has always influenced medicine, particularly in the area of reproduction; chapter 7 covers this close relationship with caesarean birth.

Chapters 8 to 15 cover the medical and surgical aspects of caesarean delivery from earliest times to current practice. The evolution of the surgical technique is covered in detail, including extraperitoneal and lower segment caesarean section through to caesarean hysterectomy. There is a detailed chapter on anaesthesia for caesarean section pointing out the early mortality with both regional and general techniques. The controversial topic of caesarean delivery by maternal choice is reviewed in appropriate detail.

The book is easy to read, like an interesting novel on the history of caesarean section. Globally millions of caesarean births are performed by thousands of obstetricians and I would urge every obstetrician to read this book and digest the true history of the procedure and its evolution to current day practice.

Sir Sabaratam Arulkumaran
Past President, British Medical Association – BMA (2013-2014)
Past President, Royal College of Obstetricians and Gynaecologists – RCOG (2007-2010)
Past President, International Federation of Gynaecology and Obstetrics – FIGO (2012-2015)

Preface

Caesarean delivery evolved from a postmortem ritual to satisfy the law and religious edicts to a last-ditch, almost always fatal, intervention in live women and from that to what is now the most commonly performed operation on women worldwide. It is one of the more dramatic surgical events, albeit a relatively simple operation in most instances. The unique component is that it directly involves two patients, and the sometimes competing interests of each of those patients has dictated how the operation has developed.

Medical practice should be viewed within the social, religious, economic and cultural framework of its time. Reading about the plight of women with obstructed labour in the 17th to 19th centuries is harrowing and hard to comprehend in the 21st century, although some women still confront similar conditions in parts of the world. How the caesarean operation safely overcame this mortal complication is a blend of tragedy, courage (mostly from the patients), innovation, art and science. Most of the advances and innovation came from detailed and cumulative case reviews - what would now be called audit.

I have tried to show the human side of the characters involved by using extensive quotations from their work. Apart from the entertaining language of the different eras, it gives the essence of their rationale and humanity. It took little more than a century for caesarean section to evolve from desperate women driven to perform the operation on themselves, to the modern woman, confident in its safety, requesting it for reasons of convenience and reduced risks of damage to herself and her baby.

T.F. Baskett
Halifax, Nova Scotia

Acknowledgements

Much of the core work for this book was done in Washington, DC during a history fellowship in 2008, granted by the American College of Obstetricians and Gynecologists (ACOG). During that fellowship, and in the years before and since, I was graciously assisted by Mary Hyde, Senior Director, ACOG Resource Centre and Debra Scarborough, Librarian and Archivist of the Jacobs History Library of ACOG – the latter's ability to track a source was uncanny and has been of great help. The following individuals have helped me: Ron Cyr of East Lansing, Michigan, not only translated Rousset's text, but helped guide me to relevant American and French articles; Tony Koller of Cape Town, in an act of great generosity, gave me his copy of Young's *Caesarean Section*; Ernesto Castelazo, Mexico City, provided me with meticulously translated articles and texts from the Mexican and Latin American literature; Eugene Pearce, Kansas City, Missouri kindly sent me a copy of Dr Manfred Thurmann's English translation of Max Sanger's monograph, *Der Kaiserschnitt*; Christoph Brezinka, Innsbruck, Austria provided me with his translation of Gaspard Bauhin's account of the early caesarean delivery in 1500. I am indebted to you all.

Over many years I have visited and used the facilities of the following libraries: the British Library, London; the Wellcome Institute for the History of Medicine, London; The Royal College of Obstetricians and Gynaecologists, London; the Royal Society of Medicine, London; the Bay Jacobs History Library of ACOG, Washington, DC; The United States National Library of Medicine, Bethesda, Maryland. At home, the staff of the Kellogg Health Sciences Library, Dalhousie University, Halifax, Nova Scotia have always been most gracious and helpful in tracking down obscure articles.

The digital image collection of the National Library of Medicine was the source of figures 3.2, 6.1, 8.5, 8.6, 8.8, 9.1, 9.3, 9.4, 10.1, 10.2, 10.3, 11.1, 11.3, 11.5, 12.1, 12.2, 14.2 and 16.2 – all in the public domain. Figure 8.7 (Robert Harris) came courtesy of the Pennsylvania Hospital Historic Collections, Philadelphia. Photography Collection Box L8.

My wife, Yvette, typed the manuscript and has supported my endeavours for more than fifty years – none of it would happen without her.

Chapter 1

Caesarean birth in folklore, legend and myth

Those who are delivered by caesarean section are in good company; two of the more notable gods, Aesculapius, God of Medicine, and Bacchus, God of Wine, were reputed to have been born in this manner. Having said that, it must be noted that Aesculapius came into the world in somewhat unsavory circumstances.[1]

His father, Apollo, upon discovering that his mortal mistress, Coronis, had been unfaithful to him kills her and while she is on her funeral pyre removes his son, Aesculapius, through a cut in her abdomen. (Figure 1.1)

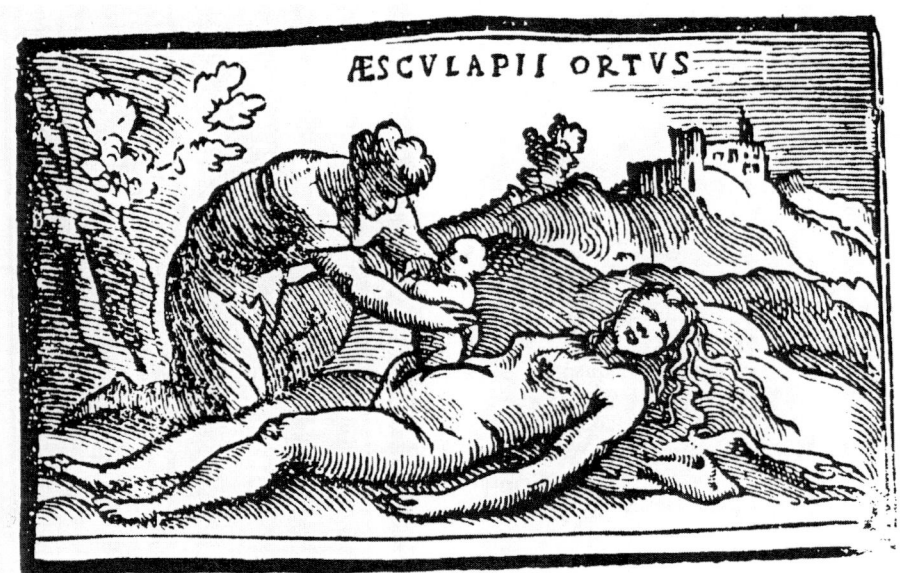

Figure 1.1 Delivery of Aesculapius by his father Apollo through an incision in the abdomen of Coronis. Woodcut from De Re Medica by Alessandro Benedetti, 1549

The upbringing of Aesculapius was entrusted to the centaur, Chiron, who taught him the art of healing and medicine.[2] Both Aesculapius and Apollo carried the title of Paen, *'the healer'*. Furthermore, through five of his goddess daughters, Aesculapius covered the spectrum of celestial healing: Hygieia (sanitation), Aceso (healing), Iaso (recuperation), Aglaea (beauty) and Panacea (universal remedy).

Bacchus had a similarly complicated background. His father was Zeus, King of the Gods no less, and his mother, Semele, was a mere mortal - albeit the daughter of King Cadmus of Thebes. This was a long story involving much deceit and myth manipulation, that ended with poor old Semele being engulfed in flames initiated by thunderbolts from Zeus. Whereupon, having second thoughts, Zeus removed the baby from her abdomen, sewed him into his own thigh, later releasing the fully-grown baby. Thus, Zeus topped Apollo's feat by adding transplantation and surrogacy to his medical achievements. To make matters worse for Aesculapius he is later slain by one of Zeus' thunderbolts, which Zeus had a habit of hurling about with abandon and not always with suitable forethought or accuracy. At any rate, Bacchus soon established his credentials as the God of Wine and, even more appropriate in an obstetrical sense, as God of nature's fertility - exemplified by the fast growing and productive grapevine. He later became legendary for extreme cavorting with a group of female devotees (Bacchantes), leading to much drunken revelry – Bacchanalia.

In Virgil's Aeneid we are told that Lichas, one of Heracles' attendants, *'had been cut out of his dead mothers womb and then made sacred .....'* (Book x, Line 315)

In Ireland, where there is no shortage of myths and legends, it is said that a caesarean delivery occurred in 200 BC[3]. Eithrie, the wife of Connor McNessa, King of Ulster, carelessly fell into the River Inny near the end of her first pregnancy. She was dead upon retrieval from the river so an immediate incision was made in her abdomen and a living son delivered. He was named Furbaidh, derived from the Gaelic word 'Urbaidh' – to cut.

According to Eastern mythology, in the sixth century BC, Queen Maha Maya, the virginal queen of King Suddhodana, had both a miraculous conception and delivery. She conceived during a dream that a great white elephant pierced her right side with one of its six white tusks. Ten months later she gave birth, through the same right flank to Siddhartha – the future Buddha. (Figure 1.2)

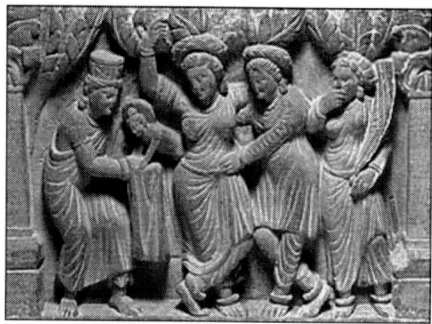

Figure 1.2 The Birth of Siddhartha (Buddha) from the flank of his mother, Queen Maha Maya

The Shahnameh or The Book of Kings is the epic compendium of Persian myths and legends. Written by the nationally revered poet Hakim Abolgasem Ferdowsi (940 – 1020 AD) it was finished in 1010 and recounted the unusual birth of Rostam.[4] The mother, Roudabeth, was greatly swollen with the large fetus and could not deliver. In despair her husband, Zal, took a feather from Simorgh (another legend, this time in the form of a bird). With Simorgh's feather as inspiration Zal put his wife to sleep with wine and asked the high priest (also part-time surgeon) to use his dagger to cut into the abdomen and uterus.[5,6]

As Ferdowsi wrote:

'The high priest slit the flank of the Goddess of Beauty (Roudabeth) and the head of the boy came into view.

The boy, Rostam, was brought out of the womb magnificently and without harm.'

The poem goes on to describe the care of the wound and the recovery of both mother and baby.

Trolle recounts the 13th century Nordic legend, *'The Saga of the Volsungs'*, in which King Rerer's wife endures a seven-year pregnancy.[7] This does seem a bit much, exceeding by far the gestation period of even the largest mammals. Unable to deliver, and quite understandably losing patience, she ordered the child to be cut from her and this was done. Reputedly the baby was a mature boy, to be named Volsung, who walked over and kissed his mother just before she died.

British royalty, always a handy source of legend, real or imagined, provided a couple of early dubious tales of abdominal delivery.

In March, 1316, Robert II, King of Scotland, was reputedly born via abdominal incision after his mother, Marjory Bruce, was severely injured falling from her horse near Paisley Abbey in late pregnancy. One of her followers performed the operation but the baby sustained an injury to one eye.[8] Throughout his life Robert was afflicted with eye inflammation, which led to his nickname King Blear-eye, later shortened to King Blearie. Doubts of authenticity of this tale include the fact that both his eyes were subject to inflammation and that there was no contemporary historical record of what would have been a momentous event, until 400 years later in 1710.[9]

The other oft-quoted royal abdominal delivery was that of Jane Seymour, the third of many ill-fated wives of Henry VIII. She gave birth to a son, Edward VI, on 12th October 1537 at Hampton Court Palace and died twelve days later.[10] Once again, the contemporary historians did not imply abdominal delivery and the first record to suggest this was almost one hundred years after the event.[9] The other myth, apparently started with malice aforethought, was the reputed response of Henry VIII when asked, as the labour became difficult, whom he would favour to survive, *'The Queen or his son?'* He supposedly answered, *'Save the life of the child for another wife can easily be found'*.

Thus, there is insufficient proof of the two royal abdominal deliveries or of Henry VIII's callous response – not that he wasn't capable of such a sentiment.

Shakespeare, of course, got into the act in his play Macbeth; first performed in 1606. As he faces the wrath of Macduff in battle at the castle on Dunsinane Hill, Macbeth clings in desperation to the prophecy of the witches' apparition *'.....for none of woman born shall harm Macbeth,'* claiming:

*'I bear a charmed life which must not yield
To one of woman born'*

His hope is trumped by Macduff who declares that his manner of birth makes him *'not of woman born'*:

*'Despair thy charm
And let the angel whom thou still hast served
Tell thee Macduff was from his mother's womb
Untimely ripped'* V.6.51-56

Whereupon Macduff slays Macbeth.

The phrase *'untimely ripped'* is generally felt to refer to a postmortem abdominal incision and those delivered in this manner were said to be *'not of woman born'*.

It is widely acknowledged that Shakespeare used the Chronicles of Holinshed as the source for part of his historical plays Macbeth, Cymbeline and King Lear. Raphael Holinshed (c1529-1580) produced the first edition of his chronicles in 1577, volume 5 of which was devoted to Scottish history.[11] In Holinshed's chronicle Macduff's words were, *'I was not born of my mother, but ripped out of her womb'*. Shakespeare used the same word *'ripped'* in his play Cymbeline, when Posthumous' mother appears in an apparition, lamenting that she was forsaken by Lucina, the Goddess of Childbirth:

*'Lucina lent not me her aid
But took me in my throes
That from me was Posthumous ripped'* V.5.137-139

So, all in all, there are many entertaining myths and legends but no solid evidence to support abdominal delivery in any of the stories.

REFERENCES

1. Hart GD. Aesculepius the God of Medicine. Royal Society of Medicine Press: London; 2000.
2. Retsas S. Gods behaving badly. J Med Biog 2015;23:14-17.
3. O'Sullivan JF. Caesarean birth. Ulster Med J 1990; 59:1-10.
4. Khatamee MA. Historical Perspective: "Rostam" is born: How? By Caesarean Section. ACOG Clin Review 2000; 5:12-16. American College of Obstetricians and Gynecologists, Washington DC.
5. Browne EG, Arabian Medicine. London: Cambridge University Press; 1921. p79.
6. Torpin R, Vafaie I. The birth of Rustam. Am J Obstet Gynecol 1961;81:185-9.
7. Trolle D. The History of Caesarean Section. Copenhagen: C.A. Reitzel Booksellers; 1982. p12.
8. Rutherford WJ. Caesarian section post-mortem in the fourteenth century. Glasgow Med J 1937;128:12-17.
9. Young JH. Caesarean Section: the History and Development of the Operation from Earliest Times. London: HK Lewis &Co Ltd;1944.
10. Clippingdale SD. The accouchement of Queen Jane Seymour. J Obstet Gynaecol Br Emp 1921;28:109-116.
11. Mason R. Scotland. In: The Oxford Handbook of Holinshed's Chronicles. Kewes P, Archer IW, Heal F.(eds). Oxford: Oxford University Press; 2013.

Chapter 2

The lexicon of caesarean birth

One of the most popular explanations of the term *'caesarean'* birth is that Julius Caesar was born by this method. It is now widely accepted that this was not the case as Caesar's mother, Aurelia, lived in apparent good health for many years after Caesar's birth – and this at a time when abdominal delivery was only carried out post mortem.

The questions that arise are, how did the cognomen (surname) Caesar arise and come to be applied to members of the Julia family or clan, and whence the legend that Julius Caesar was born in this manner?

Possibilities for the origin of the name Caesar include the following:
- Pliny the Elder (23-79 AD) wrote in his Natural History[1] that the *'first Caesar'* was so-called because he was cut from his mother's uterus: *'a caeso matris uterus'* (caeso meaning to cut).
- Children born by abdominal incision were known as caesones
- One of the children was born with long or thick hair (caesaries, a lot of hair).
- An infant born with blue-green eyes (caesius, blue-green).
- The first notable to have the cognomen Caesar was Sextus Julius Caesar who served as Praetor in the second Punic war (228-202 BC), during which he killed an elephant (caesar = elephant in the Punic language).

The manner by which the famous Roman emperor Julius Caesar (100-44 BC) became linked with caesarean birth was tortuous and has been covered in detail by Blumenfeld-Kosinski.[2] Pliny wrote that in the case of the woman's death the infant was cut from the mother's uterus:

'Those delivered when their mothers have been cut open are born under better auspices. The elder Scipio Africanus (236-183 BC) was one such, and the first of the Caesars, who owed his name to the surgery performed on his mother, the same operation which gave rise to the family name Caeso.' [1]

The translation of Pliny's sentence is ambiguous and could refer to Scipio Africanus as the first Caesar or another member of the Julia family with the surname Caesar. However, as Beagon notes, the elder Scipio Africanus was not known by the cognomen *'Caesar'*, so the first of the Caesars was a different person.[3] Furthermore, Scipio Africanus' mother also lived many years after his birth, so both of Pliny's examples of caesarean delivery seem unlikely.[4]

Pliny described humans as the creatures '*....for whose sake nature appears to have created everything else*'[1] His treatise was a cultural and natural history of the human race in the early Christian era.[3] However, sometimes his written observations were thought to be influenced more by his imagination than solid fact and Celsus, who wrote his respected book, *De Re Medica*, about 30 AD, did not mention this or any other cases of caesarean delivery. The historian, Gaius Suetonius Tranquillus (69-140 AD), wrote the biographies of The Twelve Caesars in 120 AD; however, the first section of the biography of Julius Caesar, including his birth, was lost. It was Isidore, the Bishop of Seville, (c 570-636 AD) in his *Etymologies (The Origins)* who wrote that Julius Caesar was called Caesar either because he was cut from his dead mother's uterus or because he was born with thick hair. *Faits des Romains (The Deeds of the Romans)*, written anonymously in French in the early thirteenth century and available to a wider audience, used Isidore as its source but removed any doubt by simply stating that Julius Caesar was cut from his mother's womb and that he had a lot of hair.[5,6]

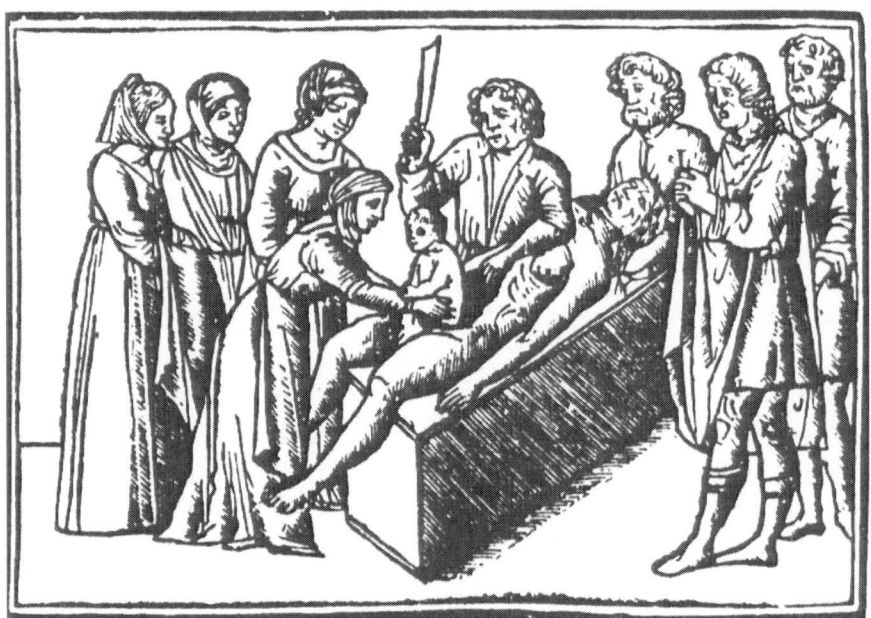

Figure 2.1
Purported birth of Julius Caesar depicted in the annotated edition of Suetonius' 'The Twelve Caesars', published by Beroaldus and Antonius in 1506. This widely distributed woodcut image helped establish the myth that Julius Caesar was born in this manner

Thus, the unconfirmed nature of Julius Caesar's birth via abdominal incision became ensconced in historical texts; in part because it was such an attractive and unusual method of birth for an exceptional emperor. In 1506 when Beroaldus and Antonius published an annotated version of *The Twelve Caesars* they included a woodcut illustration depicting the abdominal birth of Julius Caesar – further strengthening the legend. (Figure 2.1)

The cognomen Caesar, which really started as a nickname, became hereditary in the Julia family and was later adopted by the Roman emperors as a title – the first being Julius Caesar's adopted son and successor, Caesar Augustus.[7] As the word Caesar became equivalent to emperor, the caesarean operation was regarded as a great undertaking and one worthy of such a title. In the late 19th/early 20th century the Germans called the operation *'Kaiserschnitt'* when the Kaiser, the German emperor, was an important and all-powerful national figure. (Kaiser, emperor; schnitt, cut). This was followed in other countries such as Denmark (Kjsersnitt), Holland (Keizersnede), Norway (Keisersnitt) and Sweden (Kejsersnitt). Similar terms were used in Japan, Korea and the Slavic countries.

Ironically, Kaiser Wilhelm II (1859-1941), the German emperor and King of Prussia from 1888 to 1918 would probably have benefited from being born by caesarean section. He was a breech birth and his obstetrician, Eduard Martin (1809-1875), Chief of Obstetrics at the University of Berlin, was confronted with one of the undesirable complications of breech delivery - extended arms: *'I also brought down the left arm, which was extended at the side of the head, not without considerable effort because of the lack of space at the pelvic outlet.'*[8] Wilhelm was left with a permanently weak and underdeveloped left arm – obviously a severe brachial plexus injury. Furthermore, the infant *'appeared quite lifeless'* at birth and required *'half an hour of resuscitation'* - suggesting possible hypoxic brain damage.[9] There are those who felt this disability, and the ineffective corrective mechanical braces he was forced to wear as a child, distorted his view of himself in a strong masculine culture. His erratic and at times bombastic behaviour contributed to the inexorable slide into World War I. It may be a bit of an obstetrical stretch, but had Wilhelm himself been delivered by Kaiserschnitt in 1859, World War I might not have started and millions of senseless deaths been averted.

The king of Rome, Numa Pompilius (762-716 BC) established a set of rulings known collectively as *Lex Regia* (Law of Kings or Royal Law). One of these forbade the burial of a pregnant woman with her child in utero, ruling that the infant had to be cut out of her uterus before the burial of both separately. It has been postulated that as the rulers of the Roman

Empire became the Caesars, the Lex Regia became Lex Caesarea. Because this law specifically ordained postmortem abdominal delivery, along with the name of the law, Lex Caesarea, makes this one of the most plausible origins of the term caesarean delivery.[10]

The first medical text to use the term *caesarean childbirth* was written by François Rousset (c1530-1603) in 1581.[11] Written in French as *Enfantement Caesarien*, Rousset wrote in the preface: '*.....concerning the method of childbirth that I have dubbed 'Caesarean'...*' Many authors attribute the first use of the term *'caesarean section'* to the French obstetrician, Jacques Guillemeau (1550-1612), who used the term *'la section caesarienne'* in his 1609 text, *De L'Heureux Accouchement des Femmes*.[12] In fact, Rousset wrote of *'section caesarienne'* in his text in 1581 – *'De l'utilitié et necessité de ceste section caesarienne'* [11]

All of the possible Latin derivative words for caesarean (caedo, caesum) and section (seco) imply cutting. Thus, to avoid the theoretical tautology of 'cut cut' in 'caesarean section', the terms caesarean birth, caesarean delivery, or caesarean operation have been suggested.[13] That said, caesarean section remains a practical and commonly used term.

Sometime around the end of the 19th century American English dropped the use of the diphthong – the union of two vowels. This was extended to proper names, so that Caesar became Cesar. This was unfortunate as, whatever the origin of the term *'caesarean'* section, it is derived from the name or word spelt with the diphthong 'ae'. Even Caesar's Palace in Las Vegas is spelt correctly!

In the medieval era children born by caesarean section were sometimes given names to reflect their special status: Nonnatus (not born), Ingenito (unbegotten), Fortunatus (fortunate, lucky).[2] The Catalan saint, Raymond Nonnatus (1204-1240), was said to have been given his name because he was born by postmortem caesarean section. Appropriately he became the patron saint of childbirth and midwives.

REFERENCES

1. The Elder Pliny on the Human Animal. Natural History, Book 7. Translated by Mary Beagon. Oxford:Clarendon Press; 2005.
2. Blumenfeld – Kosinski R. Not of Woman Born: Representations of Caesarean Birth in Medieval and Renaissance Culture. Ithaca: Cornell University Press; 1990. p1,143-53.
3. Beagan M. Commentary in: The Elder Pliny on the Human Animal. Natural History, Book 7. Translated by Mary Beagan. Oxford: Clarendon Press; 2005 p201-7.
4. Cyr RM, Baskett TF. Caesarean Birth: the Work of François Rousset in Renaissance France. Cambridge: Cambridge University Press; 2010. p29.
5. Van Dongen PWJ. Caesarean section – etymology and early history. S Afr J Obstet Gynaecol 2009;15:62-6.
6. Barroso M. Post-mortem cesarean section and embryotomy: myth medicine and gender in Greco-Roman culture. Acta Med-Hist Adriat 2013;11:75-88.
7. Janson T. A Natural History of Latin. Oxford: Oxford University Press; 2004. p40-1.
8. Jacoby MG. The birth of Kaiser Wilhelm II (1859-1941) and his birth injury. J Med Biog 2008;16:178-83.
9. Shingleton HM. Historical perspective. Kaiser Willy: Victim of his birth injuries? ACOG Clin Review 2005;10:12-14. American College of Obstetricians and Gynecologists, Washington DC.
10. Raju TNK. The birth of Caesar and the cesarean misnomer. Am J Perinatol 2007;24:567-8.
11. Rousset F. Traitte Nouveau de L'Hysterotomotokie ou Enfantement Caesarien. Paris: Denys du Val; 1581. p1-3.
12. Guillemeau J. De L'Heureux Accouchement des Femmes. Paris: Abraham Picard;1609.
13. Cesarean Childbirth: Report of a consensus developmental conference. National Institutes of Health Pub No. 82-2067. Washington DC: US Dept Health and Human Services; 1981.

Chapter 3

Postmortem caesarean delivery

Postmortem caesarean section is probably the oldest recognised form of caesarean delivery. In addition to the entertaining, sometimes fanciful and unsubstantiated examples given in chapter 1, there are some early and more credible references to this practice.

The most commonly cited written reference to postmortem caesarean section comes from the first Roman Kingdom and its second king, Numa Pompilius (716-672 BC). One of the rulings in his *Lex Regia* (Royal Law) was as follows:

'The royal law forbids the burial of a pregnant woman before the child is extracted from the womb; who violates this law is deemed to have destroyed the child's expectancy of life along with the mother.' [1,2]

As noted in chapter 2 this law and its successive name, *Lex Caesarea* (Law of the Caesars), is one of the most plausible origins of the term 'caesarean' delivery.

There is, however, an earlier possible reference to postmortem caesarean delivery. This was included in the code of laws, the Hammurabi Code, formulated by the King of Babylon, Hammurabi (1795-1750 BC), and inscribed on cuneiform tablets; so-called because the nib used to inscribe the words on wet clay had a triangular tip, producing wedge-shaped (cuneiform) script. The laws were later transcribed onto a large basalt stone which is in the Louvre, Paris. A number of these laws applied to medicine and surgery, one of which confirmed that surgery took place in that era and that it carried a career–ending penalty for substandard practice:

'If a doctor has treated a free man with a metal knife for a severe wound, and has caused the man to die......his hands shall be cut off.' [3]

The code also contained the following legal text: *'Ibiq–iltum, the son of Sin–magir, adopted the male child pulled out of the womb, the son of the deceased woman Atkasim.'* 'Pulled out' could refer to delivery by forceps extraction or via abdominal incision, but because obstetric forceps were unknown in that era it might be interpreted that *'pulled out'* referred to caesarean section.[1,4]

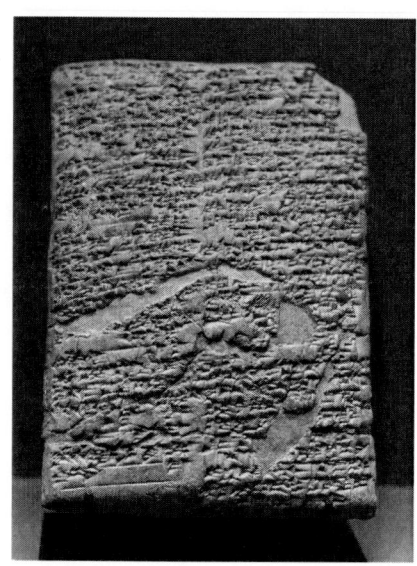

Figure 3.1 The Hammurabi Code, formulated by the King of Babylon, Hammurabi (1795-1750 BC)
In the collections of the Louvre Museum (Department of Near Eastern Antiquities)

Thus, there was written law proclaiming postmortem caesarean delivery at least 2700 years ago and possibly up to 1000 years before that.

Sushruta, who practiced in the 5th century BC is regarded as the father of Indian medicine and surgery. He documented his medical experience and knowledge in a Samhita, or compendium, which included reference to postmortem caesarean section: [5]

'A child, moving in the womb of a dead mother, who has just expired (from convulsions etc) during parturition at term, like a goat should be removed immediately by the surgeon from the womb; as delay in extracting the child may lead to its death.'

Interestingly, and confirming that there is nothing new under the sun, in the Samhita the principle of simulation training for the trainee surgeon was outlined: [6]

'In all acts connected with surgical operations of incision, etc, the pupil should be fully instructed as regards the channels along or into which the operations or applications are to be made. A pupil, otherwise well read, but uninitiated into the practice (of medicine or surgery) is not competent to take in hand the medical or surgical treatment of a disease. The art of making specific forms of incision should be taught by making cuts into the body of a gourd, watermelon or cucumber .....and suturing on pieces of cloth, skin or hide.'

The earliest obstetrical writings of Hippocrates (460-377 BC), Celsus (25 BC-73 AD) and Soranus (98-138AD) did not mention abdominal delivery in any form. Although, as physicians, they would not have been involved in postmortem abdominal delivery, it seems unlikely that they would not have recorded cases had they been aware – particularly if the infant had survived. On the other hand, operating on the dead would have been done only by non-medical lay persons. It is also likely that almost all of the cases in their era were performed well after the death of the woman and without survival of the infant. Such a demeaning occupation may have been thought unsuitable to include in a medical treatise. Furthermore, in that era, before the Christian church's edicts in the 13th century, the law may have been followed infrequently.

Just how long the practice of postmortem caesarean delivery preceded the Lex Regia of Numa Pompilius is a matter of conjecture. Observations of animal sacrifices and from hunting would have confirmed that the animal fetus in utero survived after its mother was killed. Postmortem spontaneous vaginal delivery of the fetus may have suggested that the fetus could live for many hours, and even days, after the death of the mother. These so-called *'corpse deliveries'* or *'coffin births'*, now known to be due to putrefactive gases expelling the fetus days after the death of the mother, [7] may have suggested continued fetal life in an era when the fetus was thought to play a physically active role in propelling itself to delivery. Indeed, no less an authority than William Harvey (1578-1657), the discoverer of the circulation of blood, wrote the following in the obstetrical section (De Partu) of his text on fetal development: [8]

'How great furtherance the foetus doth confere in its own birth, several observations do clearly evince. A certain woman here amongst us was, (being dead overnight) left alone in her chamber, but the next morning an infant was there found between her legs, which had by its own force wrought its release.'

Bernard of Gordon (b1258) was a physician who taught and practiced medicine at Montpellier for more than 30 years. His guide to the performance of postmortem caesarean section in his 1305 compendium *Practica Sive Lilium Medicinae* was the first in a Western medical text.

Guy de Chauliac (1298-1368) was the preeminent French surgeon of the middle ages. (Figure 3.2). He took holy orders and then studied medicine at Toulouse, Montpellier, Paris and Bologna. He spent most of his life as surgeon to three popes at Avignon.

Unlike many physicians he remained to treat patients during the epidemic of plague in 1348; he contracted the disease but survived.[9] His major opus, *Chirugia Magna* (Great Surgery) was published in 1363 which he completed, he said, *'for the solace of old age, solely for the exercise of his mind.'*

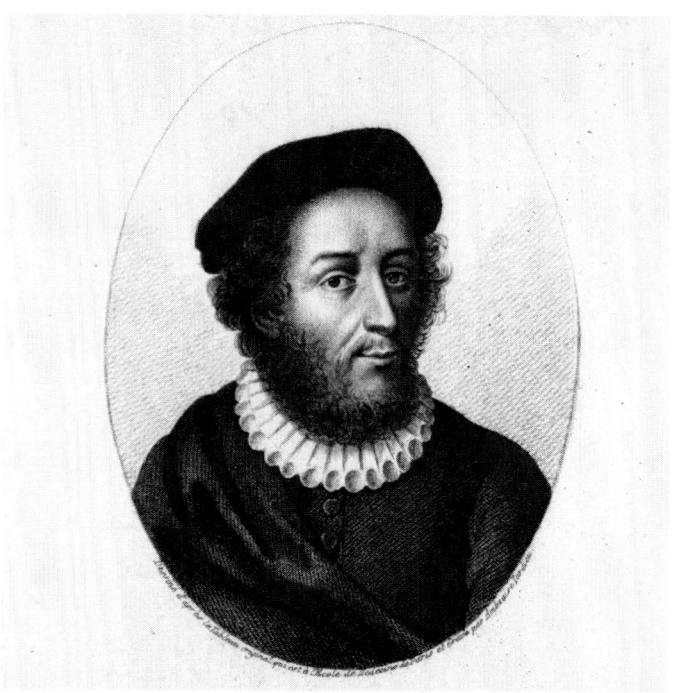

Figure 3.2
Guy de Chauliac (1298-1368), the eminent French surgeon, published his Chirurgia Magna in 1363. It was one of the earliest texts to give instructions on the performance of postmortem casarean section.

It became a standard surgical text for the next three hundred years and some eighty editions were published in seven languages.[9] One of the earliest references to postmortem caesarean delivery was in this book.[10]

'If it happens that the woman herself is dead and you suspect that the fetus is alive......Open the woman with a razor on the left side (for that part provides better access than the right because of the liver), and put in thy fingers and draw out the child.'

Attempts to prevent suffocation of the fetus after the mother's death included keeping her mouth and uterus open. Indeed, Guy de Chauliac noted this in his instructions before carrying out postmortem caesarean: *'.. the woman's mouth and uterus are held open (as women wish).....'* [10.] It can be seen, however, that he was skeptical of its efficacy as this seemed to be merely a concession to any assembled women midwives – *'as women wish.'*

The first printed textbook for midwives, *Der Swangern Frawen und Hebammen Rosengarten*, was written by Eucharius Rösslin and published in 1513. Rösslin was the city physician at Frankfurt-am-Main and responsible for supervision of the official city midwives. English translations by Richard

Jonas ('a studious and diligent clerk') and Thomas Raynold, physician, were published in 1540 and 1545 as *The Byrth of Mankynde or The Womans Booke*.[11] This book, which was the basis for most texts for midwives until the 1700s, gave instruction for postmortem caesarean section, as follows:

'If it chance that the woman in her labour die, and the child having life in it, then shall it be need to keep open the womans mouth, and also the nether places, so that the child may by that means both receive and also expel air and breath, which otherwise might be stopped to the destruction of the child. And then to turn her on the left side, and there to cut her open, and so to take out the child.' [12]

In 1708, Pierre Dionis (d. 1718) of Paris also advocated putting a gag in the dead woman's mouth for the same theoretical reason. But, like de Chauliac, he proposed this manoeuvre only to assuage the ignorance of the midwives who attended the labouring woman: [13]

'Not because I think that the child breathes in the womb as the vulgar do; who if it is found dead, which is very often the case, are sure to lay the blame on the surgeon if he has not put a gag in the mother's mouth. He must by no means omit this circumstance, for the satisfaction of those that are present and to put it out of the power of silly women and others who know nothing, to throw malicious reflections upon him.'

Barroso pointed out that the Portuguese physician, Rodrigo de Castro (1546-1627), declared in 1603 *'After the mother's death, the neonate cannot survive in the womb.....when the mother's life and her movements cease, the neonate's life and its heartbeats also cease.'* [2]

Jane Sharp, one of the most experienced and respected English midwives of the late 17th and early 18th century,[14] wrote in the 4th edition of her *Compleat Midwives Companion* in 1725 *'.....if the mother die in childbearing, and the child be alive, then you must keep the woman's mouth and privities open that the child may receive air to breathe, or it will be promptly stifled.'* She went on to write *'.....then turn the woman on her left side, and there cut her open and take out the infant.'* [15] She quoted Rodrigo de Castro, as noted above, but disagreed with him and believed the child *'.....may live a while without the mother; but the midwife must keep the womb open that it not be stifled till the surgeon cuts it out.'* [15] From these two passages the exact role of the midwife *vis-à-vis* postmortem caesarean section was unclear; on the one hand, she instructed the midwife to *'cut her open,'* but later stated that the midwife's role was to wait *'till the surgeon cuts it out.'*

Exactly when surgeons became involved with postmortem caesarean deliveries is unknown. Some of the earliest illustrations of caesarean birth in the 14th century show only women in attendance – suggesting that female midwives performed the operation. [16] One of these illustrations shows a midwife holding open the women's mouth – the recommendation that was alluded to in de Chauliac's text. By the 15th century the illustrations, most of which depict the alleged abdominal birth of Julius Caesar, shows male figures in the position of operator, [16] – such as in figure 2.1. This was about the time that female midwives increasingly began to call in male surgeon/men-midwives to avoid blame in complicated obstetric cases.[17]

The reasons for postmortem caesarean delivery of the infant varied through time:
- The law of the land: Lex Caesarea.
- Burial ritual.
- Fear that the fetus could be buried alive within its dead mother.
- Hope of rescuing the fetus alive after its mother's death.
- To baptise the infant. This became common from the 13th century through edicts of the Christian church (see chapter 7).
- The unbaptised child could not be buried in consecrated ground
- Inheritance law.

Not all authorities agreed that the woman who died undelivered should have her abdomen opened to remove the fetus. Many found this an affront to the dignity of the woman and to the sanctity of death. In 1345 the Islandic bishop, Jon Sigurdsson, issued the following decree: [18]

'It is beyond doubt that a woman who dies with the child should, like other people, be buried in the churchyard, and the child should not be cut or taken out.'

The length of time the fetus could survive after the death of its mother was the source of much speculation, and opinion varied from a few minutes to several hours. There were claims of infants being cut out alive many hours after the mother's death, but most of these were discounted. In those cases that produced a live infant, it usually survived only for a few minutes or hours: ie long enough for baptism to take place. It is probable that in many of these cases the signs of life in the infant were disputable and interpreted through the eyes of hopeful optimism, allied to the desire to achieve the much sought after baptism.

The predicament of the surgeon in this context was outlined by Pierre Dionis, who was opposed to caesarean section in the living but supported its use postmortem. (Figure 3.3). He acknowledged the difficulty in some cases of establishing with certainty the life or death of the infant, but erred on the side of baptism in doubtful cases: [13]

'That it may happen that an infant may be alive, and have a few gasping sighs to breath out, though we cannot discover any manifest pulsation of the navel-string; in which case 'twould be to fall into the fatal misfortune of

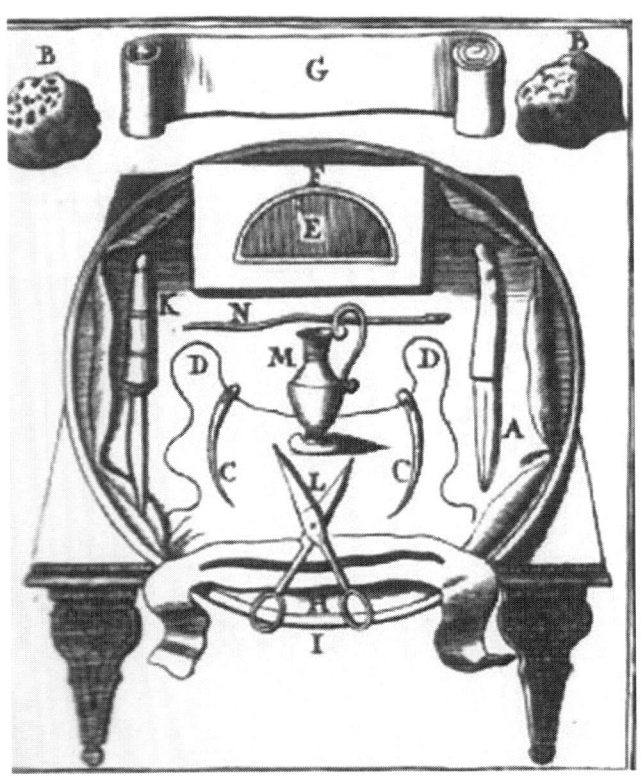

Figure 3.3
*Equipment necessary to carry out postmortem caesarean section,
according to Pierre Dionis* [13]

*refusing baptism to a living child, because not strong enough to give us any certain signs of its life. The other reason is, that in these sorts of operations the patient's chamber is always full of relations or neighbors, the most of which are intimidated and pre-possessed with the most unreasonable prejudices......
If in such cases the chirurgeon refuse to baptize the child, he will draw upon him the hatred of the publick, and none of the women will ever forgive him.'*

Certain diagnosis of the mother's death could be hard to pinpoint in the era before auscultation of either the maternal or fetal heartbeat. It was known that visible respiration could cease many minutes before the maternal heartbeat and circulation stopped. Cases were recorded in which abdominal incisions were started, only to have the woman react violently after her presumed death. Jean-Louis Baudeloque (1746-1810) recounted one such case in which a surgeon, believing the woman to be dead, opened the uterus and extracted the baby only to find her moving and complaining of his surgical assault. [19] He fled, and only with difficulty was persuaded by her relatives to return and stitch up the wound. She survived but sued, alleging surgical incompetence as she was left with a ventral hernia. Jean Astruc (1684-1766) of Paris had a more radical approach to this conundrum. *'…..before I consented to have her opened, I caused two incisions to be made in the buttocks, of a sufficient size to cause some motion, if any life remained.'* [20]

The dilemma was well summarised by Charpentier in the late 19th century. [21]

'We possess, at present, no absolute timely sign on which we may rely as pointing to the maternal death.' He pointed out that the fetus was unlikely to survive long in cases of chronic maternal disease, such as tuberculosis and typhoid fever. In such cases he wrote, *'…..we cannot hope to save the infant, because its life-supplies have not cut off suddenly, but little by little.'* The best chance of infant survival in postmortem caesarean section was with sudden death of the mother from acute haemorrhage, but even then *'The section is not likely to save the child if performed beyond fifteen to twenty minutes after the maternal death.'* [21]

Recognition of the difficulty of ascertaining death of the mother with certainty, allied to the need for speed on behalf of the fetus was shown in decrees issued by the Senate of Venice in 1608 and again in 1721. These imposed severe penalties on surgeons who did not perform the postmortem caesarean with the same diligence as they would operate on a living person. In 1757 an Austrian law proclaimed: *'The operation shall be carried out with the same care as if the woman were living.'* [19]

In 1862 Ignaz Schwarz, the Public Health Officer at Fulde, Germany, summed up the conundrum facing the surgeon: [19]

'If a man is fortunate enough to obtain a living child by the caesarean section on the dead mother, he places himself of being in the unfortunate position of being suspected of having operated on a woman in a trance or, he burdens his conscience with having waited so long for the death of the mother, that he has allowed the child to die.'

Although surgeons and midwives came to know that the chances of a live infant being procured at postmortem caesarean section were very low, the Catholic Church pushed hard for the operation to be performed promptly after the women's death. This was supported by some unrealistically optimistic claims of success. For example, the Catholic diocese in Syracuse reported that postmortem caesarean had been carried out twenty times between 1735 and 1752, and had produced a live child in all cases.[19]

In Germany, in the mid 19th century, health regions began to collect population–based data on the outcomes of postmortem caesarean deliveries. These showed a very different picture. In the Kurhessen region between 1836 and 1848 there were 336,941 deliveries. Of these, 107 were postmortem caesareans and not a single fetus was delivered alive. [22]

In comparing these figures with the more optimistic reports of the previous century Ignaz Schwarz ironically wrote: *'Have the obstetricians become more honest or less skilled?'* [22] Faced with the consistent failure to rescue infants by postmortem caesarean the German obstetricians sought and succeeded in having laws on compulsory postmortem caesarean discarded. In France similar results were reported. [22]

In 1877 an Italian study from the cities of Milan, Cremona and Venice found that in 116 cases of postmortem caesarean delivery only two infants were born alive, and they both died soon after birth.[22] The incidence of postmortem caesarean delivery in this study was very high: 1 in 400 deliveries– reflecting both the high maternal death rate and the Catholic urge to save the infant for baptism. This rate compared to the German figures of 1 in 8000 deliveries. [22]

Thus, by the 1860s, while the church continued to encourage it, the legal obligation to carry out postmortem caesarean section was removed through most of Europe. There had never been such legal requirements in Britain or the United States of America. [23]

Inheritance law also played a significant role in individual cases. In most European countries if the baby was delivered alive it would come into its mother's inheritance, and if the infant subsequently died this passed on to the father. Thus, if the woman died in pregnancy but the baby could be rescued alive by postmortem or perimortem caesarean section, then the husband would inherit through the child - otherwise the estate would go to other family members. In order to be legal the child had to be baptised and to be baptised it had to show some signs of life and be well enough developed (ie close enough to term) to be considered a legal heir.

Trolle recounted such a case in Sweden in 1360. [18] A noblewoman with a considerable estate died during labour, at which point her husband, being familiar with inheritance law, insisted upon a caesarean section. The baby was baptised in the presence of witnesses and this was certified in writing. The infant died soon after, but the King of Sweden granted the deposition and the husband inherited the estate. Another case, with similar motivation, was recorded in Italy in 1545.[24] The woman, Isabella Della Volpe, came from a prominent family in Vercelli and became mortally ill late in her first pregnancy. The cause of death was recorded as *'obstruction of the brain'*, which caused her to lose *'the power of speech three or four days before her death'* – possibly eclampsia or a stroke. Despite the fact that it took more than thirty minutes after her death to organise a barber surgeon to perform the caesarean section, four eye witnesses made written depositions that the infant was born alive, was baptised and died shortly thereafter. [24]

Francois Mauriceau (1637-1709), who was the most famous obstetrician of 17th century France, was scathing in his condemnation of caesarean section for inheritance purposes: [25]

'Tis rather to satisfy the avarice of some people, who care not much whether their wives die, provided they have a child to survive them; not so much for the sake of the children, but to inherit by them afterwards; for which cause they do easily consent to this cruel operation, which is damnable policy.'

On the other hand, the Dutch surgeon, Hendrick van Roonhuyse, noted the impact on the father of a delayed postmortem caesarean section: *'To the great grief of some fathers who may thereby lose either their illustrious name, or heir to a considerable estate or both.'* [26] No mention, however, of grief caused by loss of his wife or infant!

Perimortem caesarean section

In the 20th century individual case reports continued to describe examples of postmortem caesarean with survival of the infant. In general, however, the results were poor – with many failures tending to go unreported. At the maternity hospital in Copenhagen between 1870-1980 there were 155,270 deliveries with nine postmortem caesarean sections – 1 in 17,252 deliveries. Of the ten children (1 set of twins) there were only two survivors. [18] The dismal figures from Germany in the 19th century have already been noted.

In the last fifty years postmortem caesarean section has become a great rarity. In developed countries maternal deaths are rare and many of these occur postpartum.

Increasingly it has been realised that unless carried out within five to ten minutes of the mother's death the chances of intact infant survival are slim. [27] However, rare exceptions, with intact survival after thirty minutes, still occur. [28] By the 1980s it was observed that during cardiopulmonary resuscitation (CPR) of women in the last trimester of pregnancy, removal of the fetus by caesarean section improved the likelihood of successful resuscitation of the mother. [29,30] This is due to the reduction in uterine size, thereby removing aorto-caval compression and improving ventilation and optimal positioning of the mother for CPR. [31] Thus, if a women in the last trimester of pregnancy requires CPR the current teaching is that caesarean section should be done after four minutes of failed CPR, and this will give the best outcome for both mother and child. [32,33]

A review of three triennial Reports on Confidential Enguiries into Maternal Deaths in the United Kingdom from 1994 to 2002 showed there were 6,318,726 births over those nine years.[34] In that period there were sixty-two perimortem/postmortem caesarean sections (forty-one perimortem and twenty-one postmortem) – about one per 100,000 births. From the twenty-one postmortem caesareans all the babies were stillborn. Of the forty-one perimortem cases twenty-five were stillborn, six early neonatal deaths and ten survivors – although the long term infant morbidity was not recorded. Most of these cases occurred in hospital emergency departments, as opposed to obstetric units. [34]

From a legal standpoint the offences: mutilation of a corpse and of battery, due to lack of consent, could theoretically be brought against the person performing postmortem or perimortem caesarean section. However, it is widely held that the principle of 'emergency exception' would apply and protect against litigation; assuming the operation was carried out to benefit either the child, the mother or both – regardless of the outcome. [27,35]

REFERENCES

1. Lurie S. The changing motives of cesarean section: from the ancient world to the twenty-first century. Arch Gynecol Obstet 2005;271:281-85.
2. Barroso M. Post-mortem cesarean section and embryotomy: myth, medicine and gender in Greco-Roman culture. Acta Med-Hist Adriat 2013;11:75-88
3. Haeger K. The Illustrated History of Surgery. New York: Bell Publishing Co; 1988. p18-19.
4. Oppenheim AL. A cesarean section in the second millennium BC. J Hist Med 1960;15:292-4.
5. Bhishagratna KK. An English Translation of the Sushruta Samhita. Vol 2 Calcutta: Wilkins Press;1911.p58.
6. Bhishagratna KK. An English Translation of the Sushruta Samhita. Vol 1 Calcutta: Wilkins Press;1911. p71.
7. Schulz F, Puschel K, Tsokos M. Postmortem fetal extrusion. Forensic Sci Med Path 2005;1:273-6.
8. Harvey W. Anatomical Exercitations Concerning the Generation of Living Creatures. London: James Young;1653.
9. Major RH. Classic Descriptions of Disease. 3rd edition. Springfield: Charles C Thomas; 1945.p77.
10. Guy de Chauliac. Chirugia Magna, 1363. The Chirugie of Guy de Chauliac. Margaret S. Ogden (ed). London: Oxford University Press; 1971.
11. Radcliffe W. Milestones in Midwifery. Bristol: John Wright & Sons Ltd;1967.p6-9.
12. Rösslin E. The Byrth of Mankynde. London: Thomas Raynald;1545.p101-2. Published in: The Classics of Obstetrics and Gynecology Library. New York: Gryphon Editions;1994 (facsimile).
13. Dionis P. A General Treatise of Midwifery. Faithfully translated from the French of Monsieur Dionis. London: A. Bell;1708.
14. Aveling JH. English Midwives their History and Prospects. Reprint of 1872 edition. London: Hugh Elliott Ltd; 1967.p47-54.
15. Sharp J. The Compleat Midwife's Companion: Or the Art of Midwifery Improved.

4th edition. London: John Marshall; 1725.p120-1.
16. Blumenfield-Kosinski R. Not of Women Born: Representations of Caesarean Birth in Medieval and Renaissance Culture. Ithaca: Cornell University Press;1990. p61-90.
17. McTavish L. Blame and vindication in the early modern birthing chamber. Med Hist 2006;50:447-64.
18. Trolle D. The History of Caesarean Section. Copenhagen: C.A. Reitzell Booksellers; 1982. p22-4.
19. Young JH. Caesarean Section: The History and Development of the Operation from Earliest Times. London: HK Lewis & Co Ltd; 1944. p224-34.
20. Astruc J. Elements of Midwifery. Translated by S. Ryley. London: S. Crowder and J. Coote; 1766.p167.
21. Charpentier A. Cyclopaedia of Obstetrics and Gynaecology. Obstetric Operations: The Pathology of the Puerperium. A Practical Treatise of Obstetrics. Volume 4. Translated by E.H. Grandin. New York: William Wood and Company;1887.p233-4.
22. Schafer D. Medical practice and the law in the conflict between traditional belief and empirical evidence: post-mortem caesarean section in the nineteenth century. Med Hist 1999;43:485-501.
23. Bacon CS. Legal aspects of postmortem caesarean section. Surg Gynecol Obstet 1911;12:168-77.
24. Park K. The death of Isabella Della Volpe: four eyewitness accounts of a postmortem caesarean section in 1545. Bull Med Hist 2008;82:169-89.
25. Mauriceau F. The Diseases of Women with Child and in Child-bed. 2nd edition. English translation by Hugh Chamberlen. London: John Darby; 1683. p276.
26. Van Roonhuyse H. Medico-Chirurgical Observations. Englished out of Dutch (1662) by a careful hand. London: Moses Pitt;1676.p4.
27. Katz V, Dotters DJ, Droegemueller W. Perimortem cesarean delivery. Obstet Gynecol 1986;68:571-6.
28. Capobianco G, Balata A, Mannazzu MC et al. Perimortem cesarean delivery 30 minutes after a laboring patient jumped from a fourth-floor window: baby survives and is normal at age 4 years. Am J Obstet Gynecol 2008;198:15-16.
29. DePace NL, Betesh JS, Kotler NM. 'Postmortem' cesarean with recovery of both mother and offspring. JAMA 1982;248:971-3.
30. Marx GF. Cardiopulmonary resuscitation of late-pregnant women. Anesthesiology 1982;56:156.
31. Baskett TF. Essential Management of Obstetric Emergencies. 5th edition. Bristol: Clinical Press Ltd; 2015. p293-4.
32. Katz V, Balderston K, De Freest M. Perimortem cesarean delivery: were our assumptions correct? Am J Obstet Gynecol 2005;192:1916-21.
33. Dijkman A, Huisman CM, Smit M, et al. Cardiac arrest in pregnancy: increasing use of perimortem caesarean section due to emergency skills training? BJOG 2010;117:282-87.
34. Reports on Confidential Enquiries into Maternal Deaths in the United Kingdom. Why Mothers Die 1994-96, 1997-99, 2000-2002. London: RCOG Press; 1998, 2001, 2004.
35. Fadel HE. Postmortem and Perimortem Cesarean Section: Historical, Religious and Ethical Considerations. J Islam Med Assoc 2011;43:194-200.

Chapter 4

Self–performed caesarean section

There are a number of remarkable case reports of women performing caesarean delivery on themselves - sometimes known as auto-caesarean section. The underlying themes in these unfortunate women are obstructed labour, mental illness and attempts to conceal or destroy an illegitimate pregnancy.

The first of these documented cases occurred in 1769, but was only published much later and separately by Cawley and Moseley.[1,2] It took place in Jamaica and the women in question was an unnamed slave, ironically *'belonging to Mrs Bland, a midwife.'* She performed the caesarean with a broken butcher's knife, cutting to the left of her lower midline. The baby, who had a two inch cut on his right thigh, *'…. came out by the action of his own struggling.'* A local midwife was sent for and she cut the umbilical cord, returned it and the intestines to the abdomen and stitched the abdominal wound. A surgeon attended a few hours later and judged that some dirt had been placed in the wound. He therefore removed the stitches, washed the adjacent structures, removed the placenta and resutured the wound. The woman was very weak from loss of blood, developed a fever but eventually recovered and was back to work in six weeks. The baby *'…. came into the world healthy and strong'* but died on the 6th day of *'jaw–falling'* (presumably neonatal tetanus).

The woman, who had three previous pregnancies, *'…. all with natural and easy births'* became pregnant again two years later and apparently, *'…. attempted the same operation again; but was watched and prevented, and had a regular and proper labour.'* Thus she was thwarted from becoming the first woman to have performed two caesarean sections on herself and forced instead to have a vaginal birth after previous caesarean (VBAC). The explanation for her recourse to caesarean delivery was given as : *'She was an impatient and turbulent woman, whose violence of temper was the only cause assigned for her conduct.'*[1,2]

Another sad case was reported in 1822 by Dr Samuel McClellan from the town of Nassau in the state of New York.[3] The patient was a fourteen year old servant girl who concealed a twin pregnancy. Upon coming into labour she left the house and opened her abdomen with a razor while lying in a snow bank. The incision was L–shaped, above the umbilicus and cut through into the uterine fundus. When discovered, she had buried one infant in the snowbank that she had delivered vaginally just after she made the incision. The second twin and her intestines were protruding through the incision as she ran back to the house. The doctors who were called removed the partially extruded baby from the uterine incision, along with the placenta. The abdominal wound was stitched and she recovered without incident. The fate of the infants was not recorded, though it seems likely they did not survive. This, therefore, was the first recorded case of combined vaginal/caesarean delivery of twins.

In 1876, Dr Van Guggenberg of Bavaria was summoned at 2am to an unusual emergency: *'He found the patient laying in a miserable house, on a wretched and dirty bed, exhausted and bloodless….'*[4] A dead male infant and the placenta lay between her knees. Intestines protruded through the 3.5inch (9cm), S-shaped incision in her abdomen. Dr Guggenberg washed and replaced the intestines and sutured the abdominal incision. The patient, who had seven previous pregnancies, had on this occasion laboured on and off for three days. She developed convulsions and severe abdominal pain: *'The pain and distension became so severe that the patient determined to perform caesarean section, of which she had heard.'* She used a razor and made three strokes through the incision before entering the uterus. She recovered well, *'….. soon returned to work, and has been ever since in perfect health.'*[4]

Madigan reported a case from Britain in 1883 of a woman who *'Was not of sound mind for some four or five years previously'*[5] She had six previous normal deliveries but on this occasion decided that the *'Quickest way in which to obtain relief from her labour pains'* was to cut open her abdomen, which she did. As Dr Madigan wrote:

'On arrival I found her in bed, having with a razor laid open her abdomen and uterus and plucked out a fully grown male child. A considerable portion of intestines protruded but was uninjured. Her abdominal incision measured a trifle more than five inches, and extended from an inch above the umbilicus, perfectly straight downwards. The uterine wound engaged the upper third anterior surface and the entire fundus.'

The male infant *'lay dead in an adjoining room with the cord cut across but not ligated.'* Dr Madigan cleaned and closed the wound, *'….. the uterus was firmly contracted.'* The woman died thirty hours later from peritonitis.

In 1830, Dr Luke Barker reported a case to the New York Medical and Philosophical Society that had been under his care in 1817 when he was in England.[6] A thirty-five year old woman with four children was enduring a prolonged labour when her husband verbally chastised her for taking so long. Greatly upset, she went into a back room and with a weaver's knife made an oblique five inch incision in her lower abdomen, cutting through the uterus. When Dr Barker arrived she was '.... *To all human appearance, dead – literally drenched in her own blood.*' The placenta protruded through the wound and Barker delivered this, followed by a large but dead infant. Postoperative care included castor oil enemata, twelve leeches applied to the abdomen and an opiate. Despite the above, '...*at two o'clock in the morning, forty-one hours after operation, she breathed her last.*'

Even among the consistently unusual reported cases of self-performed caesarean section the following stands out as a exceptional combination of desperation, courage and physical endurance. The case was reported in two editions of the Lancet, two weeks apart in May 1886.[7] Part of that report by Drs Baliva and Serpieri, who attended her, follows:

'A peasant woman of Viterbo, aged twenty-three, of lymphatic temperature and short stature (one metre and forty cent.), and of delicate constitution, was in the last month of pregnancy. As her condition was talked about amongst her neighbours, and provoked the anger of members of her family and of her masters, she came to the following unheard-of determination.

At 3 a.m. on the 28th of March, as she relates, with a not very sharp kitchen knife she opened her abdomen. The wound was linear, but somewhat jagged, twelve centimetres in length, situated in the middle of the right iliac region, from a little above the level of the umbilicus downwards, and from without inwards. She penetrated with a somewhat less extensive incision into the uterus, and extracted from it a male foetus at the ninth month, weighing 1 kilogramme and 900 grammes. This foetus, before being extracted from the uterus, had received several important wounds in the thorax and abdomen, whereof it died before breathing, as was undoubtedly proved by the results of the necroscopic analysis. The head had been divided from the trunk by a circular incision at the base of the neck and precisely between the penultimate and the last cervical vertebra. The cord was detached from the placenta and the foetus. The placenta was perfectly healthy. This operation completed, the patient states that she tightly bound a bandage round her body, so as to bring the edges of the wound together and prevent the protrusion of the intestinal coils; then, having dressed herself at 5 a.m., two hours after the operation, she went into Viterbo on foot, a distance of one kilometer, and visited a married sister, to whom she said nothing of what had happened, but breakfasted with her on bread and coffee and a cup of broth. She then left the house and walked about the town for some time, in order, as he states, to show herself and to put an end to the current talk about her pregnancy. At 10 o'clock still on foot, she returned to her home in the country; on reaching it she was seized with unbearable abdominal pains, followed by violent vomiting and fainting. She quickly rallied, and, the bandage having slipped upwards, almost the whole of the small intestines protruded. It was only then (about 11 o'clock) that the father, mother, and brother became aware of the serious occurrence, and went to Viterbo for medical assistance.

We were the first to arrive on the spot at 4 p.m., the same day, thirteen hours after the incision, and six hours after the escape of the intestines. We found the patient in pain, but not so much so as might have been anticipated from the gravity of the case; she was conscious and tolerably calm. She was lying dressed on a small bed in a well-ventilated room. Without loss of time, with all possible precautions, and with the limited means at our disposal in the country, we proceeded to cleanse the intestines and to replace them in the abdominal cavity, after having emptied it of copious sero-sanguinous effusion. We were scrupulously careful to secure the utmost possible cleanliness; the wound was closed with twisted sutures, and a drainage-tube placed in its most dependent part.'

The postoperative course was relatively uncomplicated and by six weeks she was described as '.... *perfectly well and walks about.*' The report concluded with the poignant sentence, '*She is under the surveillance of the judicial authority and is receiving much sympathy from the public.*'

The above cases represent the spectrum of reasons for self-performed caesarean section. One can only imagine the level of desperation, mental instability and courage required to drive a woman to self-perform caesarean section. A common factor in the reports of obstructed labour is the lack of obstetric services. Although the first documented self performed caesarean section was in 1769, such cases may have occurred since women had access to sharp cutting instruments when, alone and in despair, they sought relief from the unrelenting pain of an obstructed labour.

The number of documented cases of self-performed caesarean section is quite small – twenty-two in a recent review.[8] However, particularly with obstructed labour, there are likely to be unreported cases in areas with limited or no maternity services. Two cases have been reported in the 21st century[9,10]

In 2004 a case report was published that took place three years earlier in a remote area of Mexico.[9] A forty year old mother of seven children had a stillbirth in her eighth pregnancy – after which she was told by a midwife that she should have had a caesarean. In her ninth pregnancy she came early into a painful labour; fearful of a repeat stillbirth she sent her eight year old son to get a sharp kitchen knife. After taking three cups of alcohol she cut into her uterus via a seven inch incision in her lower abdomen. She pulled out a male infant who cried and has since thrived. Her son went to get a '*nurse*' with basic training who replaced the extruded intestines and stitched the skin. Following this she and her infant son were transported for several hours in the back of a truck to the nearest hospital. There, the uterine and abdominal wounds were sutured. One week later she returned on the bus to her home – a circuitous twelve hour journey. When the bus arrived near her district she got off and, carrying her son on her back, walked along mountain paths for one and a half hours to her home. When asked why she chose not to remain on the bus, which was scheduled to ultimately reach her home, she replied, *'It was a short cut.'*

A recent report in July 2012 came from the Philippines where a twenty-eight year old woman in late pregnancy, who had apparently just completed a course in midwifery, opened her abdomen and uterus with a kitchen knife.[10] She was discovered by her aunt, with the dead baby lying beside her. Using a regular needle and thread she had closed her own skin incision. Her uterine and abdominal wounds were surgically closed after she was transferred to hospital. She survived.

A detailed analysis of the twenty-two cases reviewed by Szabo and Brockington[8] shows that the reports came from seventeen countries and that there was an equal number in both the 19th and 20th centuries. Other details are shown below:

The instrument used was:
- knife (9),
- razor (8),
- axe (1),
- not recorded (4).

Initial closure of the skin incision was by:
- doctor (11),
- patient herself (3),
- nurse/midwife (2),
- neighbour (1),
- daughter, age 13 yr (1),
- not recorded (4).

Of the 23 infants (1 set of twins)
- 5 lived,
- 13 died (4 from wounds inflicted at the caesarean)
- 5 unknown outcome.

Thus, in only 5/18 (27.7%) with known outcome did the infant survive.

Maternal survival was better with 15/21 (71.4%) mothers with known outcome surviving. At least three of the surviving women had successful vaginal deliveries (VBAC) in a subsequent pregnancy.

The infant and maternal survival rates were no different in the 19th or 20th centuries. As Harris reported, maternal survival of self-performed caesarean section in the 19th century was superior to physician-performed caesarean.[11] The reasons for this are discussed in the next chapter.

REFERENCES

1. Cawley T. Lond Med J 1785;6:372-3.
2. Moseley B. A Treatise on Tropical Diseases. London;1795. p108-9.
3. McClellan S. Case of self-performed caesarean section. NY Med Phys J 1822;2:40-2.
4. Von Guggenberg. Case of caesarean section performed by the patient herself. BMJ 1885;1:392-3.
5. Madigan B. Death from injuries inflicted while under delusion. Lancet 1884;1:146.
6. Barker L. The history of a case of self-performed caesarean section. NY Med J 1830;1:381-3.
7. Baliva R, Serpieri A. Extraordinary caesarean operation. Lancet 1886;1:890-1,994-5.
8. Szabo A, Brockington I. Auto-caesarean section: a review of 22 cases. Arch Womens Ment Health 2014;17:79-83.
9. Molina-Sosa A, Galvan-Espinosa H, Gabriel-Guzman J, Valle RF. Self-inflicted cesarean section with maternal and fetal survival. Int J Gynecol Obstet 2004;84:287-90.
10. Andrade JI. Docs keep close watch on woman who did C-section on self. Philippine Daily Inquirer. 6 July 2012.
11. Harris RP. Six self-inflicted cesarean operations with recovery in five cases. Am J Med Sci 1888;95:150-8.

Chapter 5

Traumatic caesarean delivery

Throughout history there have been intentional or inadvertent acts of violence associated with war that caused trauma to the abdominal wall of pregnant women, resulting in the 'caesarean' delivery of infants – some of whom survived. Others, as Young reported, amounted to war crimes in the era when towns and cities were taken in battle and soldiers, ordered to massacre the citizens, used their swords to kill women and open their pregnant abdomens.[1] Other, more bizarre cases of 'collateral damage' have been reported. During the Austrian War of Succession in 1747, at the Siege of Bergen op Zoom, Netherlands, a soldier's wife was stooping over a stream to collect water when she was cut in two at the level of the uterine fundus by an errant cannonball. A nearby soldier noticed something moving in the water which, on close inspection, proved to be a living infant within its intact amniotic sac. The child was baptised, *'Albertus Ambrosius'*, and lived for several days.[2] Cases of assault with knives and accidental falls onto sharp implements or fencing not uncommonly result in penetrating wounds of the abdominal wall and uterus. These are rarely extensive enough to cause caesarean delivery and are often surprisingly well tolerated by mother and baby.[3]

A modern and grotesque form of traumatic caesarean section is that associated with newborn kidnapping.[4] These caesarean section murders are usually perpetrated by women with forensic psychopathology trying to fulfill a childbearing fantasy or to save a failing childless relationship. They befriend or stalk a woman in late pregnancy, murder her and cut out the baby from her abdomen – claiming the child as their own.[4]

Cattle horn caesarean section

As long as humans have lived in close proximity to horned animals they have been vulnerable to cattle horn injury, and none more than the pregnant woman with her protuberant abdomen and reduced mobility.

The earliest recorded and most cited case is that which occurred at Zaandam, Netherlands in 1647. A courageous woman, in the last month of pregnancy, went to the aid of her farmer husband who had been gored by an irate bull. Turning its attention to her, she was:

'Tossed a story high into the air, and her belly torn open in the assault. The fetus escaped with the secundines from the wound in the abdomen, and lay fallen in a damp and remote place.' [5]

The baby was rescued, baptised, cared for and survived. The farmer and his wife both died of their wounds. The event was commemorated in an engraving (Figure 5.1) that hung in the nearby protestant church, which came to be called Bullekerk (Bull Church).[5] Unrelated to this event in any way is the fact that, in 1971, Zaandam was the site of the first McDonalds restaurant in Europe.

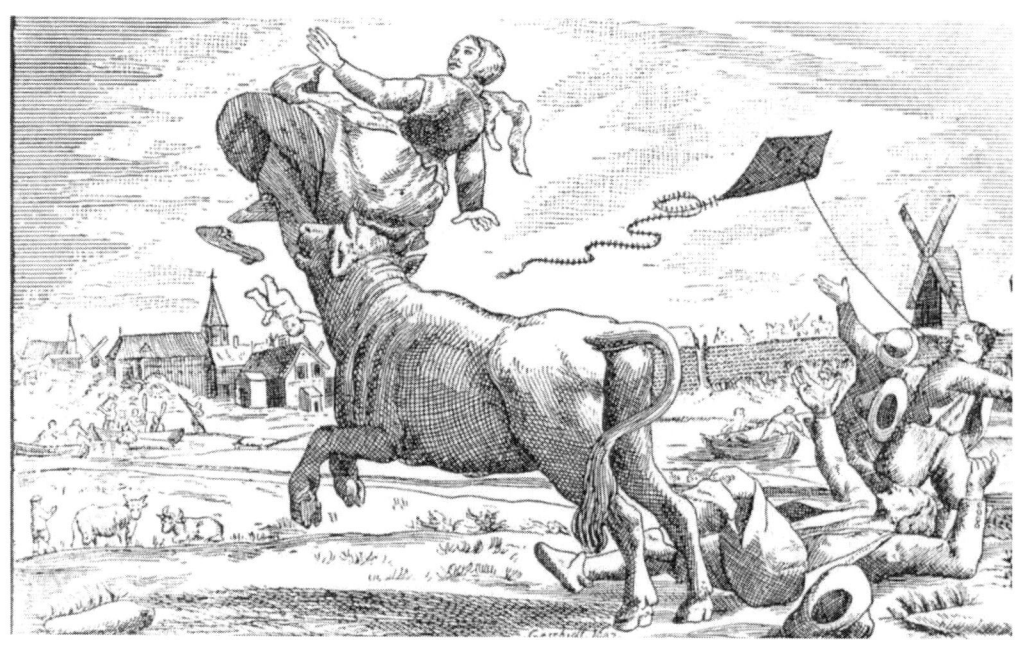

Figure 5.1
A cattle horn caesarean section.
Zaandam, 1647

A remarkable case occurred in rural Mexico in 1830. A mother of three children sat down to the routine milking of a cow when, with a sudden twist of its horned head, it ripped open her abdomen and uterus. This caused the immediate expulsion of a baby boy, who was named Liberado (the liberated) and lived to be fifty years old. When her distressed daughters came to her assistance; she instructed them to get brandy, needle and thread. Whereupon she washed the wound with the brandy, stitched the abdominal wound and walked into the house.

She was said to ..... *'live in good circumstances, and was remarkable for her masculine character and fortitude.'* Her follow up performance included three more pregnancies with normal births – making her one of an exclusive group of women in the VBACHC movement (Vaginal birth after cattle horn caesarean).[6]

Other isolated cases of cattle horn caesarean sections were reported,[7-11] and these were collated and the outcomes analysed by Robert Harris (1822-1899) an obstetrician in Philadelphia.[6] In the last quarter of the nineteenth century, Harris turned his attention to the outcome of caesarean section of all types – medical, self-performed and traumatic. His results of maternal survival after various types of caesarean section were startling. Up to 1887, over forty-nine years in New York City, only two out of eleven(18.2%) mothers survived physician-performed caesarean section and for the country as a whole, over seven years, the maternal survival was five in twenty-seven (18.5%).[5] In contrast, five of six (83.3%) woman survived self-performed caesarean section[12] and ten of fourteen (71.4%) lived after cattle horn caesareans. The corresponding figures for survival of the baby in these 19th century series were: cattle horn (55.6%), physician (37.0%) and self-performed (22.2%).[6-12] These figures are presented as maternal and perinatal mortality outcome in the table below:

Type of Caesarean	*Maternal Mortality*	*Perinatal Mortality*
Self-performed	16.7%	77.8%
Cattle horn	28.6%	44.4%
Physician- performed	81.5%	63.0%

Thus, in the United States in the 1890s, if one adhered to the published evidence-based medicine on maternal survival, you would choose first to perform caesarean section on yourself, with the second choice being your local horned animal and only as a last, and very distant resort, would you choose a physician.

Apart from the obvious aesthetic and other practical drawbacks, there was an underlying flaw in this argument that became the central theme of Harris' papers on the subject. His contention was that it was not the surgical aspects of the caesarean operation that was the main risk, rather it was the condition of the woman when she underwent the procedure that determined the outcome. Harris observed that most women whose caesarean was self-performed or carried out by cattle horn were healthy at the time the caesarean wound occurred. In contrast, medical caesareans were only performed as a last resort, often after traumatic failed efforts at vaginal delivery and with the women already exhausted, dehydrated, infected and moribund- so that her death was almost inevitable. Harris therefore wrote:

'The caesarean operation should not be regarded per se as a very dangerous procedure, and should not be held in the dread with which it was long contemplated....' [6]

Harris described what he felt was the *'abdominal and uterine tolerance'* to the incision – whether it be by surgeon, self-performed or cattle-horn. He contrasted the ability of the healthy uterus to contract after incision with that of the exhausted, infected, labouring uterus – the contraction being necessary to stop the bleeding and limit the egress of infected fluid from the uterus to the peritoneal cavity.[6]

Observation of his obstetrical colleagues in Philadelphia, and the more recent favourable results from Austria and Germany, led him to the conclusion that the optimum time to carry out caesarean section was *'shortly before labour, or as soon as possible after it had begun'*. [6]

Harris' careful work and documentation had a considerable effect in changing the timing of caesarean section away from a procedure of last resort. Ironically, he was in some ways echoing the message of François Rousset 300 years earlier (see chapter 8).

REFERENCES

1. Young JH. Caesarean Section: the History and Development of the Operation from Earliest Times. London: HK Lewis and Co Ltd; 1944. p18.
2. Burton J. An Essay Towards a Complete New System of Midwifery, Theoretical and Practical. London: James Hodges; 1751. p72-3.
3. Wright CH, Posner AC, Gilchrist J. Penetrating wounds of the gravid uterus. Am J Obstet Gynecol 1954;67:1085-90.
4. Burgess AW, Baker T, Nahirmy C, Rabun JB. Newborn kidnapping by cesarean section. J Forensic Sci 2002;47:827-30.
5. Harris RP. Cattle-horn lacerations of the abdomen and uterus in pregnant women. Am J Obstet Dis Women Child 1887;20:673-85.
6. Harris RP. Abdominal and uterine tolerance in pregnant women, as shown by the low rate of mortality under severe lacerated and other wounds as the result of direct violence. NY Obstet Gynaecol 1894;93:111-6.
7. Fritse FA. Case of a woman who, after having been gored in the abdomen by an ox in the sixth month of pregnancy, underwent the caesarean operation. London Med J 1790;11:146-160.

8. Marsh EJ. A remarkable case of penetrating and lacerated wound of the abdomen and uterus of a pregnant woman. Med Record 1867;2:148.
9. Harris RP. A tenth cattle-horn cesarean case, with recovery of the woman. Am J Dis Women Child 1887;20:1033-6.
10. Semeleder F. An additional case of cattle-horn laceration of the pregnant uterus. Am J Obstet Dis Women Child 1887;20:1036-8.
11. Morse WB. Cesarean section performed by a cow. JAMA 1906;55:1192.
12. Harris RP. Six self-inflicted cesarean operations with recovery in five cases. Am J Med Sci 1888;95:150-8.

Chapter 6

Caesarean delivery by lay persons

Some of the earliest caesarean deliveries were done by lay people, indeed they were among the first to achieve survival of the mother and child with this operation.

The first and most oft-cited case was that involving Jakob Nufer and his wife in 1500, but which was only recorded in 1586 by Gaspard Bauhin (1560-1624) a physician of Basle, Switzerland. In 1577, when Bauhin was a medical student he heard the story of a seventy-seven year old man who had recently died and who had been born by caesarean section. Intrigued, Bauhin recorded what he could find out about the case – although verification of the legendary event was not possible. In 1586, he added this account, the only record of the case, as an appendix to his Latin translation of Francois Rousset's Treatise on Caesarean Birth. This was published as part of Bauhin's *Gynaeciorum*, a three-volume compendium of works on obstetrics and gynaecology from Greek, Roman and other European sources.[1,2] (Figure 6.1)

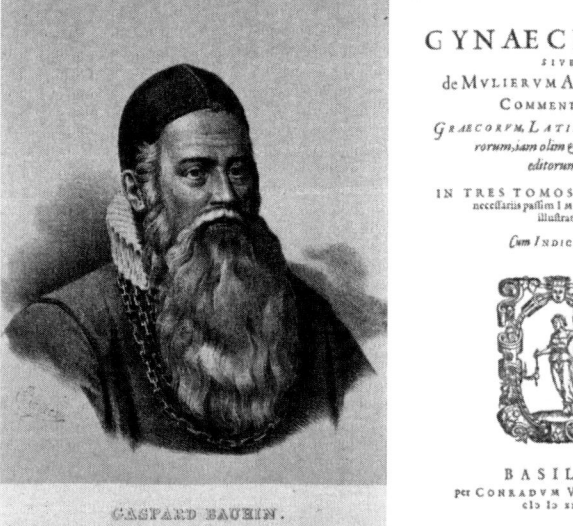

Figure 6.1 Gaspard Bauhin (1560-1624) produced a Latin translation of Roussets's 'Hysterotomotokie' as part of his compendium, 'Gynaeciorum', published in 1586. As an appendix to this work he provided the first written account of Jakob Nufer's abdominal delivery of his wife in 1500.

Jakob Nufer was a pig and rooster gelder in Siegershausen, Switzerland. His wife, Elizabeth, was expecting her first child and was in labour for several days without relief. Thirteen midwives and several barber-surgeons were consulted, but they *'could neither deliver the child nor could all these people she had called ease her pain or help her in any other way.'* [1] In desperation her husband, calling upon his skills as a sow gelder, proposed to deliver her by cutting through her abdomen, to which she readily agreed. He went to Frauenfeld, two hours distant on horseback, to get permission from the local mayor – who at first refused. Nufer persisted; the mayor relented and gave his consent. Upon his return Nufer cleared the room of midwives unless they, now informed of his plan, *'were of a hearty and fearless disposition;'* only two of the thirteen midwives felt they had these qualities and the other eleven left the room. Placing his wife on a table and calling for divine aid Nufer proceeded with a razor[1]:

'The first cut was so fortunate and well-placed that it was possible to take the child out whole and unhurt.'

The baby cried, was healthy and lived seventy-seven years, *'The child was cleaned and the wound was stuck together and closed in the way that old shoes are being stitched.'* Elizabeth Nufer recovered and in the ensuing years delivered five pregnancies in the normal way – including one set of twins.

There are a number of uncertainties about this case, including why it was first reported eighty-six years after it occurred. There are those who doubt its authenticity - fabricated tales of heroic and legendary childbirth scenes were not uncommon in those days.[3] In addition, as it was recorded, there are many features that suggest this may have been an advanced extrauterine abdominal pregnancy. If it had been an intrauterine pregnancy it is likely that after several days of obstructed labour the baby would have been stillborn and Elizabeth Nufer badly infected at the time of the caesarean section – neither of which was the case. In addition, had this been a prolonged obstructed labour due to a small pelvis Frau Nufer would not have had subsequent normal vaginal deliveries. Furthermore, the description of the *'first cut'* allowing complete delivery of the baby and with no mention of bleeding implies that the uterine wall was not incised. Thus, although not conclusive, the description and outcome support the diagnosis of advanced extrauterine pregnancy, if indeed it ever took place.[3,4]

There is a street, Jakob Nufer Strasse, in Siegershausen named to mark this event – though perhaps his wife, Elizabeth, should have received equal billing.

I include the next case in the category of lay-performed caesareans as it was carried out by an *'illiterate woman'*, albeit one who was '*.... eminent among the common people for extracting dead births....*' [5]

In January, 1738 Alice O'Neal of Charlemont, County Tyrone in the North of Ireland was in dire straits. The mother of several children and wife of a poor farmer she had been in labour for many days without respite, and all attempts to deliver her now dead baby by the local midwives had been unsuccessful. It was time to call in Mary Donally. As the local surgeon, Duncan Stewart, later recorded:[5]

'Alice O'Neal, aged about thirty-three years .... Took her labour pains, but could not be delivered of her child by several women who attempted it. She remained in this condition twelve days: the child was judged to be dead after the third day. Mary Donally, an illiterate woman, but eminent among the common people for extracting dead births, being then called, tried also to deliver her in the common way: And her attempts not succeeding, performed the Caesarean Operation. By cutting with a razor first the containing parts of the abdomen, and then the uterus; at the aperature of which she took out the child and secundines. The upper part of the incision was an inch higher, and to a side of the navel, and was continued about six inches downwards in the middle betwixt the right os ilium and the linea alba. She held the lips of the wound together with her hand, till one went a mile and returned with silk and the common needles which taylors use: with these she joined the lips in the manner of the stitch employed ordinarily for the hare-lip, and dressed the wound with whites of eggs, as she told me some days after, when led by curiosity I visited the poor woman who had undergone the operation. The cure was completed with salves of the midwife's own compounding.

In about twenty days, the patient was able to walk a mile on foot, and came to me in a farmer's house, where she showed me the wound covered with a cicatrice.'

After some minor medical ministrations from Dr Stewart, Mrs O'Neal enjoyed good health and frequently walked six miles to the nearby market town of Dungannon. This was the first caesarean section in Britain or Ireland with survival of the mother. Indeed it, would be more than fifty years before the next caesarean section with maternal survival took place in Britain.[6]

Robert Felkin (1853-1926), was an Englishman from Wolverhampton who studied medicine at Edinburgh University. Although he ultimately completed his degree he interrupted his studies after two years to undertake two trips to Africa between 1878 and 1881 – having been inspired to do so by a meeting with the explorer David Livingstone.[7] In January 1884 he presented an entertaining account of his observations on obstetric practices in Africa before the Edinburgh Obstetrical Society.[8] The published presentation is full of detailed descriptions of labour practice in Africa, interspersed with whimsical observations of his travels such as:

'One evening after a large day's march of some twenty-five miles through swamp and jungle, I was smoking my pipe before a good fire in the near proximity of a native village in the Bari district ..... Presently, however, toms-toms were beaten in the village, the sound of which produced not a little commotion .....My dragoman (who I suspect, had been enjoying a little flirtation in the village) came and asked me if I should like to see a woman cut open.' [8]

Felkin went with his dragoman (guide/interpreter) and found an elderly man with *'an ugly-looking knife'* preparing to cut open the pregnant woman's abdomen – she having been in labour for two days. Felkin persuaded them (with a gift of cloth and beads) to allow him to examine her and determined that she could safely be delivered with forceps – which he happened to have in his luggage. This he did and successfully delivered a *'very fine boy into the world.'* Presumably every travelling medical student of that era packed obstetric forceps in his first aid kit.

Felkin observed that *'labours are by no means so very easy in this part of the world, and are certainly not the painless, pleasurable affairs which some writers would have us believe.'* He was informed that in most parts of Central Africa if the woman could not be delivered vaginally, both she and her baby would perish. The exception was Uganda, *'.....the only country in Central Africa where abdominal section is practiced with the hope of saving both mother and child.'* Felkin described one such case that he observed in 1879 at Kahura (figure 6.2). [8]

'The patient was a fine healthy looking young woman of about twenty years of age. This was her first pregnancy. I was not permitted to examine her, and only entered the hut just as the operation was about to begin. The woman lay upon an inclined bed, the head of which was placed against the side of the hut. She was liberally supplied with banana wine, and was in a state of semi-intoxication. She was perfectly naked.

A band of mbugu or bark cloth fastened her thorax to the bed, another band of cloth fastened down her thighs, and a man held her ankles. Another man, standing on her right side, steadied her abdomen. The operator stood, as I entered the hut, on her left side, holding his knife aloft with his right hand, and muttering an incantation. This being done, he washed his hands and the patient's abdomen, first with banana wine and then with water. Then, having uttered a shrill cry, which was taken up by a small crowd assembled outside the hut, he proceeded to make a rapid cut in the middle line, commencing a little above the pubes, and ending just below the umbilicus. The whole

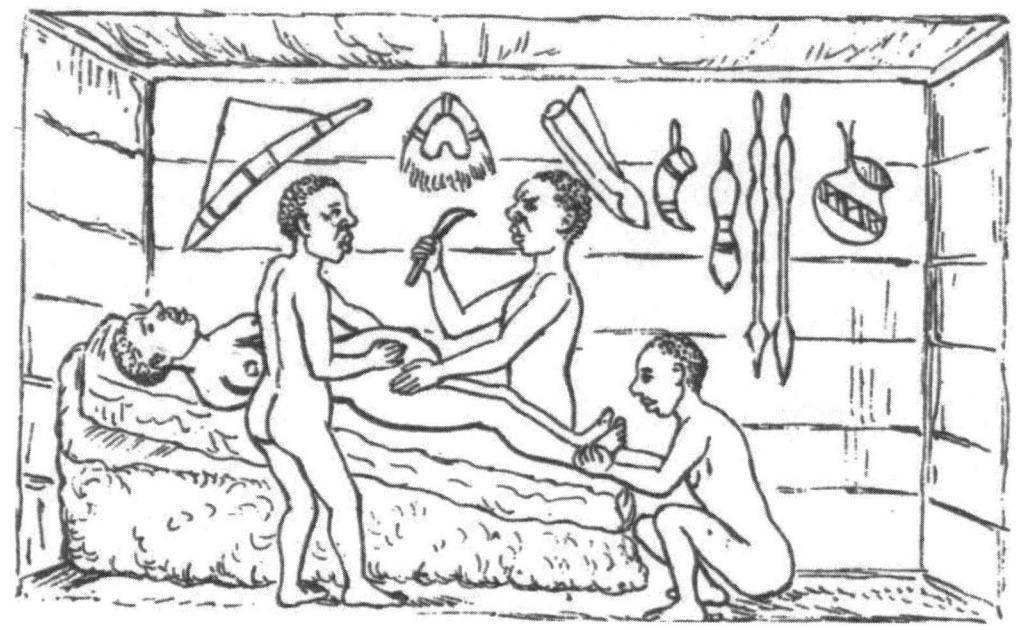

Figure 6.2 Sketch of the caesarean section in Uganda, witnessed by Robert Felkin in 1879. (From reference 8)

abdominal wall and part of the uterine wall were severed by this incision, and the liquor amnii escaped; a few bleeding-points in the abdominal wall were touched with a red-hot iron by an assistant. The operator next rapidly finished the incision in the uterine wall; his assistant held the abdominal walls apart with both hands, and as soon as the uterine wall was divided he hooked it up also with two fingers. The child was next rapidly removed, and given to another assistant after the cord had been cut, and then the operator, dropping his knife, seized the contracting uterus with both hands and gave it a squeeze or two. He next put his right hand into the uterine cavity through the incision, and with two or three fingers dilated the cervix uteri from within outwards. He then cleared the uterus of clots and the placenta, which had by this time become detached, removing it through the abdominal wound. His assistant endeavoured, but not very successfully, to prevent the escape of the intestines through the wound. The red-hot iron was next used to check some further haemorrhage from the abdominal wound, but I noticed that it was very sparingly applied. All this time the chief "surgeon" was keeping up firm pressure on the uterus, which he continued to do till it was firmly contracted. No sutures were put into the uterine wall…… The edges of the wound, i.e., the peritoneum, were brought into close apposition, seven thin iron spikes, well polished, like acupressure needles, being used for the purpose, and fastened by string made from bark cloth. A paste prepared by chewing two different roots and spitting the pulp into a bowl was then thickly plastered over the wound, a banana leaf warmed over the fire being placed on the top of that, and, finally, a firm bandage of mbugu cloth completed the operation..'

One notes the number of relatively sophisticated components of this operation; attention to haemostasis with cautery and the knowledge that the uterus must be made to contract to avoid uterine haemorrhage. A dominant theme throughout was the use of liberal quantities of banana wine; serving as a partial anaesthetic for the suffering woman, as well as antisepsis for the knife, abdominal wall and the hands of the operator. Felkin remained in the area for eleven days and observed her mostly uneventful recovery, as well as that of the baby.

For how long these caesarean sections had been carried out in this area of Africa is unknown, but it was clearly a well practiced routine in 1879.

REFERENCES

1. Bauhin G. Francisci Rousseti. De Partu Caesareo tractatus. In: Gynaeciorum Sive de Mulerium Affectibus Commentarii. Basle:Conrad Vualdkirch; 1586.
2. Cyr RM, Baskett TF. Caesarean Birth: the Work of Francois Rousset in Renaissance France. Cambridge: Cambridge University Press; 2008. p3-4.
3. Pickrell KL. An inquiry into the history of cesarean section. Bull Soc Hist Med 1935;4:414-53.
4. Trolle D. The History of Caesarean Section. Copenhagen: C.A Reitzel Booksellers; 1982. p29.
5. Stewart D. The caesarean operation done with success by a midwife. Edin Med Essays Observ 1742;5:439-41.
6. Naqui NH. James Barlow (1767-1839): operator of the first successful caesarean section in England. BJOG 1985;92:468-72.
7. Dunn PM. Perinatal lessons from the past. Robert Felkin MD (1853-1926) and caesarean delivery in Central Africa (1879). Arch Dis Child Fetal Neonatal Ed 1999;80:F 250-1.
8. Felkin RW. Notes on labour in Central Africa. Edin Med J 1884;29:922-30.

Chapter 7

Religion and caesarean birth

Religion has long played a role in the disease and suffering of humankind. Illness and catastrophic events were attributed to the wrath of various deities, and not until the Hippocratic epoch was illness and disease separated from divine displeasure. Notwithstanding, divine guidance continued to be invoked in medical texts up to the modern era. Even now many patients and their relatives will seek celestial assistance in combating ill health; during my training in 1960s Ireland it was not uncommon for them to offer the exhortation, *'May God guide your hands'*, before a surgical procedure.

Religious belief in the past was partly shaped by fear of evil spirits, including the spirits of the dead. In this context the fetus was seen in some cultures – the Maori New Zealanders and the Galician Jews – as a potential malign influence after the death of its mother.[1] Thus, cutting out the fetus and separate burial of the mother and her infant was considered essential to avoid such consequences.

For many centuries organised religion has and continues to proclaim rules aimed at regulating the sexuality and reproductive choices of women. In relation to caesarean delivery this was most pronounced in the latter half of the second millennium.

Judaism

The Mishna is a written collection of oral laws compiled in the 2nd century BC from the Rabbinical teachings of the previous four centuries. This was incorporated into the Talmud – the authoritative compendium of Jewish law. Most of the references to caesarean delivery come from the older, Mishna portion of the Talmud.

There is reference to *Yotze dophen*, which, coming from the words *Yotze*, go out, leave, and *dophen*, wall, flank, has been interpreted as being born through the abdominal wall or via caesarean section.[2,3] Animals born by caesarean section (*Yotze dophen*) for sacrifice or ritual slaughter are specifically mentioned in the Talmud and there is one reference to an animal which survived caesarean section and had a subsequent vaginal delivery (VBAC).[2] One could interpret another statement as evidence of VBAC in humans; the relevant passage reads: *'Neither a Yotze dophen nor its successor can receive the rights of primogeniture......'*[2,4,5] The fact that there was a successor implied recovery from the caesarean section and a subsequent pregnancy. Another written law suggesting maternal survival after caesarean delivery was, *'In the case of Yotze dophen, we do not observe either the days of ritual uncleanness or the days of purification.'*[2,3,4]

Thus, these descriptions, albeit implicit rather than explicit, could reasonably be interpreted as caesarean deliveries with expected survival of the mother and infant. However, there are no concomitant medical commentaries to support this. It has been pointed out that the Talmud articles of law could just be theoretical, as there was a tendency to cover all eventualities, however unlikely.[2] Another possible confounder is that the retrospective interpretation of these laws may be biased by modern surgical knowledge, unknown at the time of the original oral and written compilation. On the other hand, caesarean delivery with survival of the mother may have been common enough not to warrant special mention in the Talmund, beyond the legal aspects.[2,4]

That postmortem caesarean section was performed in the days of the Mishna was suggested by specific reference to this procedure in the dying, labouring woman, even on the Sabbath: *'If a woman was in labour and died on the Sabbath, a knife is brought, her abdomen opened, and the child extracted.'*[3,4] What is possible, but not certain, was that during that same era, more than 2000 years ago, the Jews were performing caesarean section on living women with maternal and infant survival.

In later centuries, when the debate of craniotomy versus caesarean section became relevant, reference to the Talmud supported destructive procedures on the fetus to save the mother in obstructed labour.[4,6] *'The woman who was having difficulty in bearing – the fetus is cut up and withdrawn piece by piece, the parent's life taking precedence over the fetus's life......'.*[6]

Roman Catholic Church

By the 13th century Roman Catholicism was the dominant religion in Western Europe and its Church Courts claimed authority over a wide range of human affairs. At the heart of the church's approach to caesarean delivery was the Christian doctrine of *'original sin'* by Adam and Eve; which stated that every infant entering the world was imbued with this sin which could only be removed by baptism. Otherwise, according to St Augustine, the infant's immortal soul was condemned to eternal damnation. The church's position was softened in the 13th century when it was decided that the soul of unbaptised infants went to a form of limbo and might be saved by God's mercy. Nonetheless, to the believer, lack of baptism was a very serious omission. Apparently the first church official to recommend postmortem caesarean section to achieve baptism of a potentially surviving infant was the Archbishop of Paris, Odon de Sully (1196-1258).[7] This was emphasised by the influential Thomas Aquinas (1225-1274), who was also responsible for stressing the church's opposition to any form of contraception.[8]

Neonatal baptism was so important that even non-Catholics were encouraged to perform this rite, so-called *'heretic baptism'*. This was considered valid provided it was carried out in the name of the holy Trinity. Furthermore, holy water was not necessary, any water would do. This was endorsed by the Council of Trent, an important Catholic ecumenical council held in Trento and Bologna over an eighteen year period (1545-1563). Many of us outside the church have performed this ritual and brought a degree of comfort to distressed parents.

Although Thomas Aquinas had taught that intrauterine baptism was invalid, this was later accepted by many Catholic scholars, and a number of cunning syringe-like devices were invented for this purpose.[9] Paul Portal (1630-1703), an obstetrician at the Hôtel Dieu, Paris advised pre-emptive baptism in the case of delivery of a footling breech: *'If the feet of the child come foremost, you must take care to baptise them immediately'*.[10]

In the early Middle Ages medicine was controlled by those in religious orders. In France the Catholic Church established hospitals, Les Hôtel Dieu, throughout the country, starting in the 7th century. The nurses were untrained Sisters of Charity who provided care as a religious duty. These hospitals were only taken over and run by the municipal authorities from the middle of the 16th century. The most famous was the Hôtel Dieu in Paris, situated close to Notre Dame Cathedral, which became the premier obstetric teaching hospital in France for midwives, physicians and surgeons. By the 12th century the church discouraged priests from personal involvement in the practice of medicine.[7] The performance of caesarean section was left to midwives and eventually ceded to surgeons. A major role for priests was to ensure that postmortem caesarean section was carried out for baptismal purposes, and this was emphasised in the licencing of midwives, which was controlled by the Church's courts.[11,12] A 15th century English manual outlined the duties of the parish priest towards the midwife in the event of a woman's death in childbirth:[11]

> *'For to undo her with a knife*
> *And for to save the child's life*
> *And see that it christened be*
> *For that is a deed of charity.'*

However, if there was no other qualified person present at a woman's death in childbirth, the priest could perform the postmortem caesarean.[13] Although postmortem caesarean section had been encouraged by the church since the 1200s its performance was relatively rare.[14] Stimulated by the church a number of authorities passed laws making postmortem caesarean section a legal requirement, including Venice (1608), Austria (1757) and Frankfurt (1768); most of these laws also emphasised that the operation should be carried out with the same care as if the women were alive.

In 1745, Father Francesco Emanuello Cangiamila (1702-1763), a Sicilian priest, published his *Embriologia Sacra* (Sacred Embryology), which was to have a strong influence on the promotion of postmortem caesarean section in Catholic European countries and their colonies.[14-17] This work gave detailed advice to priests on baptism of the miscarried fetus and how to perform caesarean section in order to baptise the infant. Charles VII of Sicily was so inspired by this work that he issued a decree in 1749 making the operation compulsory on any woman who died during pregnancy, and imposing the death penalty on those who failed to fulfill this duty.[14,15] In 1759 the same king occupied the Spanish throne as Charles III and distributed a copy of his Sicilian law to the Spanish bishops.[14] *Embriologia Sacra* was translated into Spanish by Father Jose Manuel Rodriguez and was circulated to the bishops of Mexico by the Viceroy in 1772, along with a directive to encourage postmortem caesarean section to achieve baptism.[16,17] In turn, the Bishop of Mexico sent an edict to the priests informing them that due to the dearth of surgeons in many areas they would have to take up the task: '*.....it is our will that all of the priests purchase and have at home the small book by Father Jose Rodriguez in which is explained the manner in which the operation is performed comfortably and easily, in order for such priests to do it by themselves.....*'[16] In many South American countries priests were actively recruited and encouraged by the church to perform postmortem caesarean section.[14,15]

In 1733 a group of physicians in Paris asked the Doctors of Theology of the University of Paris to rule on whether the mother or child should be sacrificed to save the other. The response confirmed that the mother could not be deliberately sacrificed to save the infant; thus, if a caesarean would always be mortal for the woman but potentially save the infant, it should not be done. On the other hand, in obstructed labour, if the mother's life could be saved by craniotomy and piecemeal vaginal delivery of the fetus, it should not be done. This was the main reason that caesarean delivery was more common in Catholic countries, as craniotomy on a living fetus was forbidden. Thus, in the context of the most common obstetric conundrum of obstructed labour - the infant was given precedence over the mother, to whom the alternative, caesarean section, was almost always fatal.[18] However, in 1811, Napoleon, Emperor of France, was willing to go against this ruling during the difficult first labour of his wife, Empress Marie-Louise. He was asked by the accoucheur, Antoine Dubois, whom should he chose to save if such a decision became necessary; Napoleon replied, *'Treat the Empress as you would a shopkeeper's wife in Rue St Martin, but if one life must be lost, by all means save the mother.'*[19] As it turned out Dubois was able to safely deliver the son, Napoleon II, without lethal operative intervention.

Islam

The religion of Islam was founded in the 7th century and by the 8th century the Islamic empire extended from Bagdad, Iraq to Cordoba in Spain. As they conquered new territory they also absorbed the local scholarly traditions and knowledge; one of Muhammad's declarations being: *'The ink of scholars is more precious than the blood of martyrs'*. They therefore kept a close working relationship with Jewish and Indian scholars, and all the classic Greek, Roman, Jewish and Hindu texts, including the Sushruta, were translated into Arabic.[20] Thus, they would have been aware of the tradition of postmortem caesarean delivery.

Albiruni (973-1048) was an important Islamic history and philosophy scholar. In one of his books on the history of nations (c1000) he included reference to the supposed birth of one of the Caesars by postmortem caesarean section. A 1307 manuscript of this book contains an illustration of caesarean delivery, as does a later manuscript of Ferdowsi's Book of Kings , describing the legendary caesarean birth of Rostam (see chapter 1).[20,21] This has been taken as evidence that caesarean delivery was carried out by Arab surgeons,[21,22] However, descriptions of miraculous birth to help create legendary characters were not unusual in antiquity and cannot be taken as proof of caesarean delivery.[23] Furthermore, the influential surgical text by Albucasis (936-1013), the renowned surgeon from Cordoba, provides great detail on obstetric operations, including delivery of the fetus by destructive techniques – but no mention of caesarean section.[24] There is no reference to caesarean delivery in the Koran.[20] It has been suggested that the surgical texts, copied from earlier civilisations, were more theoretical and not actually put into practice.[23]

One error, in the otherwise excellent book by Young,[25] stated that caesarean delivery was forbidden among Muslims: *'Mohammedanism absolutely forbids caesarean section......'*. This has since been comprehensively disproven.[20-22,24] It seems, that in 1863, a Dr Rique of the French Army was given this incorrect information by a supposed Islamist authority, who turned out to be nothing of the kind.[20] He published this misinformation in the medical literature[26] and it was subsequently quoted by Young and others.[25,27] Recent reviews have confirmed that postmortem caesarean delivery was permitted in Islam and may have been carried out in the middle ages by Arab surgeons.[20-22,24]

Hinduism

The obstetrical practice of the Hindus was derived from the Sushrata Samhita outlined in chapter 3. This included postmortem caesarean section and craniotomy with fetal dismemberment in obstructed labour.[28]

REFERENCES

1. Ela A. Fear of the fetus: an ancient cause for the cesarean section. Am J Obstet Gynecol 1922;3:445-8.
2. Boss J. The antiquity of caesarean section with maternal survival: the Jewish tradition. Med Hist 1961;5:117-31.
3. Lurie S, Mamet Y, "Yotzeh dofen": cesarean section in the days of the Mishna and Talmud. Isr J Obstet Gynecol 2001;12:111-3.
4. Preuss J. Biblical and Talmudic Medicine. London: Jason Aronson Inc; 1993.p420-31.
5. Lurie S. Vaginal delivery after cesarean delivery in the days of the Talmud. Vesalius 2006;12:23-4.
6. Guttmacher AF. Traditional Judaism and birth control. Judaism 1967;16:159-65.
7. Blumenfeld-Kosinski R. Not of Woman Born: Representations of Caesarean Birth in Medieval and Renaissance Culture. Ithaca: Cornell University Press;1990. p24-27.
8. Baskett TF. The Pill and the Pope. West Engl Med J, 2016, 115 No 3 Article 7, 1-14
9. Hibbard B. The Obstetrician's Armentarium. San Anselmo, California: Norman Publishing; 2000. p219.
10. Portal P. The Complete Practice of Men and Women Midwives: Or, the True Manner of Assisting a Woman in Child-Bearing. (English translation from

the original, 1685). London: J Johnston;1763.p23.
11. Donnison J. Midwives and Medical Men. Hong Kong: Historical Publication Ltd; 1988. p15-17.
12. Evenden D. The Midwives of Seventeenth-Century London. Cambridge: Cambridge University Press; 2000. p24-30.
13. Savona-Ventura C. The influence of the Roman Catholic Church on midwifery practice in Malta. Med Hist 1995;39:18-34.
14. Rigau-Perez JG. Surgery at the service of theology: postmortem cesarean sections in Puerto Rico and the Royal Cedula of 1804. Hispanic Am Hist Rev 1995;75:377-404.
15. Warren A. An operation for evangelization: Friar Francisco Gonzalez Laguna, the cesarean section, and fetal baptism in late colonial Peru. Bull Hist Med 2009;83:647-75.
16. Castelazo AL History of Gynecology and Obstetrics in Mexico. Monograph: Mexican Federation of Obstetrics and Gynecology; 1970.
17. Uribe-Elias R. The cesarean operation in Mexico. In: Viesca T (ed). Historia de la Medicina en Mexico. Universidad Nacional Autonoma de Mexico: Mexico;2007.p299-311.
18. Ryan JG. The chapel and the operating room: the struggle of Roman Catholic clergy, physicians, and believers with the dilemmas of obstetric surgery, 1800-1900. Bull Hist Med 2002;76:461-94.
19. Cameron M. On the relief of labour with impaction by abdominal section, as a substitute for the performance of craniotomy. BMJ 1891;1:509-13.
20. Naqvi NH. Caesarean section in early Islamic literature. Saudi Med J 1986;7:21-5.
21. Al Fallouji M. Arabic caesarian section: Islamic history and current practice. Scot Med J 1993;38:30.
22. Fadel HE. Postmortem and perimortem cesarean section: historical, religious and ethical considerations. J Islam Med Assoc 2011;43:194-200.
23. Savage-Smith E. The practice of surgery in Islamic lands: myth and reality. Soc Hist Med 2000;13:307-321.
24. Fadel HE. Obstetrics in Islamic medicine: an historical perspective. J Islam Med Assoc 1996;28:114-9.
25. Young JH. Caesarean Section: the History and Development of the Operation from Earliest Times. London: HK Lewis and Co Ltd;1944.p7.
26. Rique C. Etudes sur la medicine legale ches les Arabes. Gaz Med Paris 1863;3:156-162.
27. Wright St Clair RE. Historical aspects of caesarean section. NZ Med J 1963;62:409-412.
28. Findley P. Priests of Lucina: The Story of Obstetrics. Boston: Little Brown and Company; 1939.p22

Chapter 8

Development of medically performed caesarean section

The operation performed by Jakob Nufer in 1500 and outlined in chapter six, whether it was a caesarean section or a laparotomy for advanced abdominal pregnancy, is usually cited as the first attempted caesarean section on a living woman, There were a few other reports of caesarean delivery by surgeons in the early 16th century, but none with any stamp of authenticity.[1]

Early texts on caesarean delivery

The first physician to advocate caesarean section on a living woman was François Rousset (c 1530-1603) in 1581. Not only that, he did so in a text devoted solely to the subject: *Traitte Nouveau de L'Hysterotomotokie ou Enfantement Caesarien* (A New Treatise on Hysterotomotokie or Caesarean Childbirth).[2] (Figure 8.1)

He summarised the gist of the text in the subtitle. *'The extraction of a child through a lateral incision of the abdomen and uterus of a pregnant woman who cannot deliver by other means. And this without compromising the life of either or preventing subsequent pregnancy.'*[3] In the preface Rousset wrote of his reasons for proposing and promoting caesarean delivery, using the dramatic language of the day:[3]

'I was finally brought to this point by the sight of suffering, worry, terror, and supplication – the pitiful look on the faces of these poor creatures suffering through a living Hell, crying murder, and pleading with us, hands joined in prayer, to provide them with whatever assistance we might.'

François Rousset was born in Pithiviers, France and studied medicine in Paris and Montpellier, getting his medical degree from the latter university. As he gained experience his reputation grew and he was called upon to attend ancient and noble families and ultimately was appointed physician to the king, Henry IV.

TRAITTE
NOVVEAV DE
l'*Hysterotomotokie*,
OV
Enfantement Cæsarien.

QVI EST

Extraction de l'enfant par incision laterale du vētre, & matrice de la femme grosse ne pouuant autrement accoucher. Et ce sans preiudicier à la vie de l'vn, ny de l'autre; ny empescher la fœcondité maternelle par aprés.

PAR
Françoys Rousset Medecin.

A PARIS,

Chez Denys du Val, au cheual volant, rue S. Iean de Beauuais.

M. D. LXXXI.

Auec priuilege du Roy.

Figure 8.1
Title page of Rousset's Hysterotomotokie (1581)- the first text on caesarean delivery

Rousset was a physician, 'Médicin', rather than a surgeon and the difference between the two was substantial in that era.³ Physicians were usually university educated and tended to be diagnosticians and consultants; they sometimes advised, but did not perform surgical procedures. Surgeons served practical apprenticeships and learned the surgical management – mostly of farming injuries and battlefield trauma. They drained abscesses, cut for bladder stones, set fractures and amputated limbs – the latter being the main surgical pastime in war. Surgeons did not usually have a classical education and therefore did not speak or understand Latin, the accepted and working language of the church and academics - which served to maintain ignorance among the general populace. Rousset originally wrote his text in Latin but decided first to publish a shorter edition in French. He outlined his rationale for this approach in the preface:

'To please the many French surgeons with little or no command of Latin who have been urging me to share this information with them, I have included in this abbreviated French version most of the principal points of the original - not wanting to delay the life-saving and urgent help that women reduced to this last resort may require (as happens when all other solutions have failed.)' ³

In 1583, Melchior Sebezius, of Silesia published a German translation,⁴ and in 1586, Gaspard Bauhin (1560-1624) of Basle, Switzerland produced his Latin translation.⁵

Rousset's own *'expanded Latin translation'* was published in 1590.⁶ It wasn't until 2010 that Ronald Cyr, the Canadian obstetrician and medical historian, produced an English translation of this seminal work.³ The educated English speaking obstetrician or historian up until the 20th century would have been able to read Rousset in one or all of the existing French, German or Latin editions. By the 20th century most would not be sufficiently fluent in any of these languages to fully understand the text. Hence the impetus for an English edition more than 400 years after the original.³

Rousset's book was published in 1581, but there had obviously been attempts before this by surgeons in France to deliver living women by caesarean section. Ambroise Paré (1510-1590), the premier surgeon in France of that era, had published, in 1579, his surgical treatise in which he strongly criticised the caesarean operation: *'.....which thing no man can persuade me can be done without the death of the mother.....I would never advise such a procedure where there is so much risk without any hope at all.'*⁷ He did, however, acknowledge that a successful case, which took place in 1542, had been reported to him from a trusted source, but he regarded this *'.....as a true miracle of nature.'* ⁸

Rousset included ten case histories: four from *'reliable observers'* and six *'that I can vouch for personally.'* One woman was said to have been delivered six times by caesarean, only to succumb in her seventh pregnancy after her original surgeon had died and none could be found willing to perform the operation. The same fate befell another woman delivered successfully by caesarean section in her first pregnancy, but unable to find a surgeon to deliver her second, *'…..mother and child endured a miserable death.'*[3] All the other women survived. Of the infants: two were intrauterine deaths, in one the outcome was not recorded and the rest lived.

It is clear Rousset did not perform the operation himself and that he regarded this as the domain of the surgeons. He wrote, *'I have myself recommended the performance of several such operations,'* and yet in only one of the case reports is it clear that he was consulted and then he could not attend the operation he had advised *'…..having taken to my bed with a serious illness.'*[3] On the other hand, in the section *'A short guide to surgeons on the technique of caesarean'*, Rousset's description of the operation is detailed and plausible, suggesting that he was familiar with the procedure. At this time the limited experience of caesarean delivery was that it was almost always fatal to the mother, so Rousset's claim of such a high maternal survival stretched the credulity of most observers.[9] It seems Rousset only included successful cases and there is no doubt he exaggerated the safety and simplicity of the operation. In his later Latin expanded edition he added a further five successful cases and emphasised the relative ease of the operation by pointing out that in one of these cases the surgeon was inebriated: *'If the operation succeeded with him when drunk, what may he not expect who performs it when sober, according to the justest rules of his art.'* [6,8]

The response to Rousset's book from the medical establishment of the day was negative and ranged from considered opposition to vitriolic attack. The approach of Ambroise Paré to caesarean delivery has been noted, although he did act as one of two witnesses to the cautious endorsement of Rousset's text by Henri de Monauthueil, Dean of the Faculty of Medicine at the University of Paris.[3] Jacques Guillemeau (c1550-1613), a pupil of Paré, and also surgeon to Henry IV, had done two caesareans himself and observed three others carried out by *'…..excellent surgeons and men of great experience and practice…..nevertheless of the five women on whom this has been practiced, not one hath escaped.'*[10] The most vituperative attack came from the Parisian surgeon, Jacques Marchant, who openly disputed the truth of the case reports, declared that all caesarean operations were fatal to the mother and referred to Rousset as a *'decrepit old man.'* [3,9]

In 1590 Rousset responded to these criticisms with the publication of *Dialogus Apologeticus Pro Caesareo*.[11] He included the following fetal indications for caesarean delivery: *'excessive fetal size'*, locked twins, fetal malformations, and malpresentations that could not be delivered vaginally. Among the maternal reasons were tumours and scarring from abscesses that obstructed the birth canal; he did not specifically describe contracted pelvis, but did note the maternal indication *'she may be built too narrow.'* [3] In fact, five of the ten case histories of caesarean section were followed by normal vaginal delivery in subsequent pregnancies – so contracted pelvis was not common in his series.[3]

François Rousset was the first physician to have the courage to defy the medical status quo and promote caesarean delivery of living women. His text was a remarkable blend of case reports supported by logical reasoning – Young described it as *'a masterpiece.'*[8] Rousset advised caesarean section if the woman *'…..cannot be delivered using easier or more common methods, and it becomes apparent that the mother will otherwise die undelivered'*; he also emphasised the need to perform the caesarean before the woman was *'…..exhausted and beyond hope…..'*[3] On this latter point he was far ahead of his time, and it would be 300 years before Harris and others ultimately persuaded medical opinion that the high caesarean mortality was mainly due to delaying the operation until the woman was in *articulo mortis*.[12]

The next medical text to recommend caesarean delivery came from Scipio Mercurio (1540-1616). He was born in Rome and studied medicine in Bologna and Padua, after which he spent time as a monk in the Dominican Monastery at Milan. He soon tired of monkish pursuits and returned to medicine, with a special interest in obstetrics. His book entitled *La Commare O Riccoglitrice* was written in the Roman dialect, published in 1596 and used to instruct midwives and surgeons.[13] He devoted two chapters to caesarean section and was the first to recommend this for cases of contracted pelvis: [8,13,14]

'When the fetus is extraordinarily strong, the passage narrow, the pubic bone flat, it is more than necessary to perform this operation because there is no other way out.'

Mercurio may have carried out caesarean sections himself and he reported two women he had met who underwent the operation with success near Toulouse. In whimsical mode, and perhaps to help popularise the procedure, he said the operation was as common in France as bleeding was for headache in Italy. [13,14] Mercurio gave detailed instructions how to perform the operation and advised two positions for the patient: *'one, if she is strong and courageous; the other if she is weak or afraid'* [13] (Figures 8.2 and 8.3).

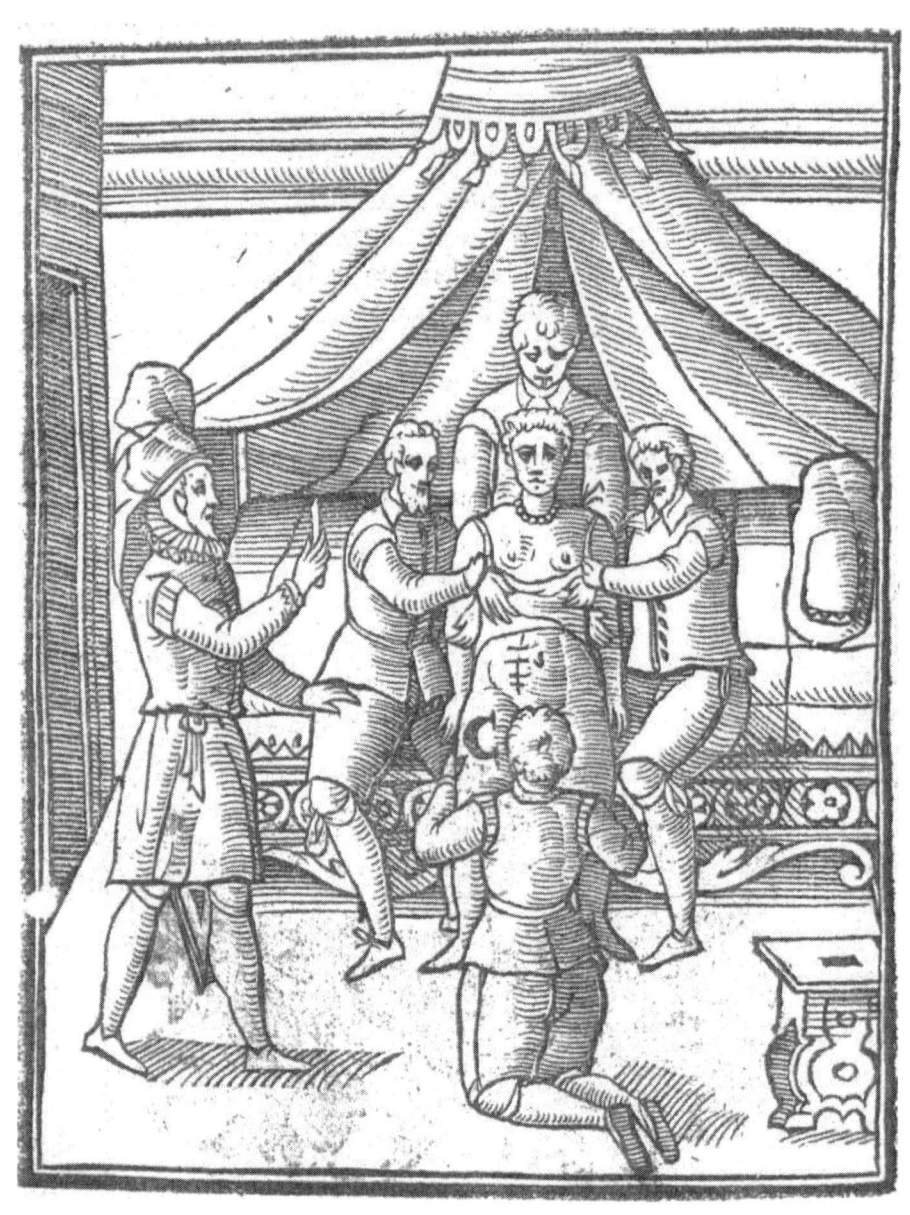

Figure 8.2
The position advised by Mercurio if the woman is '...strong and courageous.'
'Four unflinching youths or maidens are supposed to help the operator.'
The line of the incision (the outer border of the rectus abdominis muscle) and the cross-lines for suture placement were marked with ink. (From reference 13)

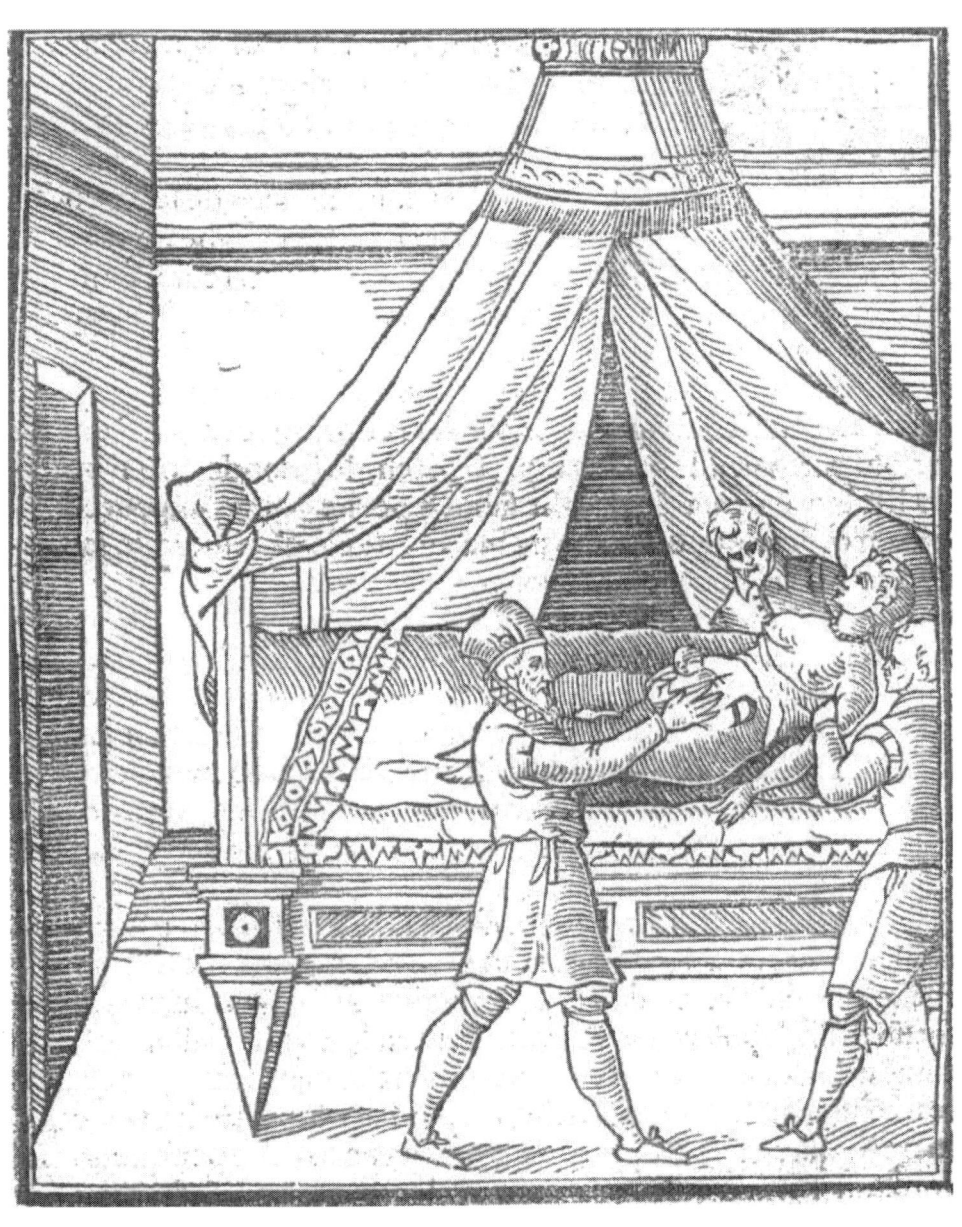

Figure 8.2
The position advised by Mercurio if the woman is '…weak or afraid.'

The book was very popular and went through a total of twenty editions and forty reprints over the next two hundred years. Whereas Rousset's French and Latin editions were never reprinted; which might explain why Mercurio's book is often cited as the first to advocate caesarean section in living women – although Mercurio clearly mentioned Rousset's work.[3,9]

In 1637, Theophilus Raynaud (1587-1663), a Jesuit priest and would-be physician, published his book *De Ortu Infantium Contra Naturam Per Sectionem Caesarean*, in which he described three successful cases from trusted sources in France. [1,8,15]

First documented medical caesarean section

The first clearly authenticated case of caesarean section in a living woman with a live intrauterine fetus took place in Wittenberg, Germany on 21st April 1610. The surgeon was Jeremias Trautmann (d 1637) and the witness who recorded the operation was Daniel Sennert (1572-1637), Professor of Medicine at Wittenberg. [1,8,16] The woman had a large, traumatic ventral hernia into which the gravid uterus had become impacted, making vaginal delivery impossible. When labour began, *'the gracious help of God was first of all implored'*, and Trautmann operated assisted by two other surgeons. Also present were two midwives, *'several honourable women'* and the Archdeacon of the local parish church – the latter presumably to ensure the appropriate concentration of divine assistance. The abdomen and uterus were each opened with a longitudinal incision, *'In fact, as soon as a way was opened, the child itself, which was healthy and unhurt, as it were by its own exertion sought the outlet'*. [1,8] The bleeding was not excessive and the stoic unanaesthetised patient claimed the pain was quite bearable. The uterus was not sutured and left protruding from the abdominal incision, which was partially sutured. By three weeks the uterus had involuted but just before its scheduled closure and replacement the woman died – twenty-five days after the operation. The infant was healthy and survived. [1,8,16]

Opposition to caesarean delivery

Up until the mid 19th century the majority of medical opinion was opposed to caesarean section, other than postmortem. In addition to the already noted opposition of Paré and Guillemeau the following were representative of the prevailing medical authority:

Percival Willoughby (1596-1685), of London and Derby, was one of the earliest English surgeons to concentrate his practice on obstetrics.[16] He worked closely with midwives and his book, Observations in Midwifery, written in the 17th century, was only published 100 years later.[17] His attitude to caesarean section reflected the English approach of his era:

'Caesarean section hath proved unprofitable to several in whose hands the women have perished and it is not used in England. I therefore pass over it in silence.'

François Mauriceau (1639-1709), the influential Parisian obstetric teacher, was completely opposed to caesarean section in living women:[18]

'But I do not know that there was ever any law, Christian or Civil, which doth ordain the martyring and killing the mother, to save the child.'

Furthermore, he expressed disbelief at the reports of successful caesarean deliveries in live women. *'If one should examine well the beginning of all the stories of this operation.....they would be found to be mere fables, and that which Rousset reports of his caesarean labours, is nothing but the ravings, capriciousness and imposture of their authors.'*[18]

Pierre Dionis, the Parisian surgeon and accoucheur, was unequivocal in his condemnation:[19]

'It is evident that the operation is by no means to be performed until the woman is dead; and those who are so bold as to venture upon it while she's alive, deserve to be severely punished for butchering her in this manner.'

Fielding Ould (1710-1789), from Galway in Ireland, studied medicine in Dublin and Paris – settling into obstetric practice in Dublin.[16] His book, A Treatise of Midwifery in Three Parts, was one of the early obstetric texts in English. In the preface he wrote:[20]

'I have taken upon me absolutely to explode the caesarean operation as repugnant not only to all the rules of theory and practice but even of humanity.'

He regarded Rousset's case reports as no more than *'fable and imposture'* and described the operation as a *'detestable, barbarous, illegal piece of inhumanity.'*[20]

Incidence of caesarean delivery in the 18th and 19th centuries

Some idea of the rarity of caesarean section in midwifery and obstetric practice can be found in the few available hospital and regional statistics of the time:[21]

So rare was the procedure that many of the experienced obstetricians whose texts were widely published had themselves not carried out the operation, or even seen it done. One such author was Robert Lee (1793-1877), a Scot who practiced at St George's Hospital, London. In the

Hospital/Region	Period	Number of deliveries	Number of Caesarean sections	Outcome
Hôpital La Maternité, Paris	1797-1811	22,000	2 caesarean sections. (1 in 11,000)	Both died
Duchy of Nassau, Germany	1821-1843	311,409	11 caesarean sections. (1 in 28,309)	10 of 11 died
Denmark	1813-1876	2,841,085	9 caesarean sections. (1 in 315,676)	8 of 9 died.

1844 edition of his Lectures on the Theory and Practice of Midwifery he wrote: [22]

'Having already defined, as clearly as I possibly can, the cases of difficult labour in which it is justifiable to employ this method of delivery, I have nothing further to say on the subject. I have never seen the operation performed on the living body.'

Some who had not performed or seen a caesarean section included a chapter on caesarean delivery in their books and acknowledged that this was based on the work of others who had. These included William Dewees and Thomas Denman.[23,24] Other texts did not even mention caesarean delivery as an option, including those by such notables as William Gifford (1734)[25] and Edmund Chapman (1759)[26] in England, and Samuel Bard (1807)[27] in the United States.

In America, Howard Kelly presented a successful case of caesarean section from Philadelphia in 1888, and noted that the last caesarean with maternal survival in that city was fifty-one years earlier.[28] Of the active members of the American Gynecological Society in 1891, only twenty-one of seventy had ever done or seen a caesarean section.[28]

The Obstetrical Society of London

Another window into the prevalence of caesarean section is available from study of the reports of the Obstetrical Society of London, which was founded after an inaugural meeting on 16th December 1858 at the Freemasons Tavern in London. The group included physicians and surgeons who devoted most of their clinical practice to obstetrics and they met to establish the society *'To advance knowledge of obstetrics and the diseases of woman and children.'* This was the first specialist obstetric society in Great

Britain, although an earlier, short-lived attempt had been made in 1825.[29] The first official meeting of the society was held on 5th January 1859, at 53 Berners Street, London and Edward Rigby, Junior (1804-1860), was elected president. The society met each month, except during the summer months of August and September.

Transactions of each meeting were published and I have reviewed these annual publications from 1859 to 1884, except for two unavailable years (1861 and 1876). The rarity of caesarean delivery in Britain in the mid to latter part of the 19th century can be gleaned from these transactions. During the twenty-four years reviewed there were 658 papers or case reports, of which only eleven (1.7%) concerned caesarean delivery – the first being in 1864.[30] Two of the early papers, presented in 1859, covered the statistics of large private midwifery practices by Robert Dunn, FRCS, and HW Bailey, FRCS, respectively.[31] Dunn reported his twenty years practice from 1831-1850 of 4049 cases with twenty-seven maternal deaths, ten craniotomies and no caesarean sections. Bailey's paper included his fifty years of practice from 1808 to 1858 of 6476 cases with none delivered by caesarean. The Obstetrical Society of London was incorporated into the Royal Society of Medicine in 1907.

Mortality with caesarean delivery in the 18th and 19th centuries

Carl Kayser (1811-1870), Professor of Statistics at Copenhagen, collected all the published cases in Europe and found only a modest fall in maternal mortality over ninety years: 1750-1800 (68%), 1801-1839 (59%). [32]

Many of these figures have been collated by Trolle[21] and are listed in the table below.

City / Country	Years (No of C/S)	Maternal mortality (%)
European literature [32]	1750 – 1800 (117)	68
	1801 – 1839 (221)	59
Paris [21]	1787 – 1876 (na)	100
Vienna [21]	1789 – 1876 (na)	100
Edinburgh [33]	1737 – 1820 (8)	100
Britain and Ireland [34]	1738 – 1880 (77)	86
Sweden [21]	1758 – 1875 (13)	100
Norway [21]	1843 – 1875 (12)	100
United States [12]	1838 – 1878 (100)	60

C/S = caesarean section   na = not available

The above figures show that *vis a vis* maternal death the pessimism of the medical establishment was thoroughly justified. It was also felt that where the mortality figures were lower it might have been due to underreporting of fatal cases.

When perinatal mortality figures were recorded, which was uncommon, the results were better, but hardly stellar: In Britain figures were of the order 37 to 41% survival.[8,33,34] Furthermore, the long term outcome of the infants, beyond initial survival or death, was rarely recorded. In 1863 the French obstetrician, Paulin Cazeaux (1808-1862), summed up this dilemma, ie: the acceptance of a high maternal death rate in part because of the expectation of a good infant outcome:

'.....but can you aver that more than a moiety of the children you save by gastrotomy will live long enough to dry the tears shed over their birth?' [35]

Contracted pelvis

From the 17th century contracted pelvis was the *bête noire* of the midwife and obstetrician, and by far the most common cause of obstructed labour. In addition to the rare causes of pelvic narrowing such as congenital deformity (Naegele's and Robert's pelves[16]), traumatic fractures or bone tumours, there were two conditions that caused the majority of cases of contracted pelvis. These were childhood rickets and the adult form of the same disease, osteomalacia – also known as malacosteon or mollities ossium (soft bone). Rickets affected infants and young children and was due to deficiency of Vitamin D; often caused by a combination of poor nutrition, excessive swaddling, keeping children inside and limited access to sunshine in the industrial slums. After the initial insult there might be catch-up growth in some, so the young adult appeared of normal stature.[36] However, the pelvic diameters were permanently narrowed so that feto-pelvic disproportion was manifest in the first and all subsequent pregnancies. Osteomalacia was due to dietary calcium deficiency, often worsened by repeated pregnancies, and leading to progressive decalcification and softening of the bones which would bend out of shape. Thus, these women might have normal early pregnancies and deliveries, only to develop feto-pelvic disproportion in subsequent labours. The softening of the bones could result in dramatic distortion of the spine and pelvic bones. The end result was a twisted, narrowed pelvic inlet with forward projection of the sacrum, the lateral pelvic walls pushed inwards and beaking of the pubic bone (Figure 8.4).

The hip and spinal deformation could cause the woman to be virtually immobilised and lose more than 40cm in height.[37] Thus, when one delves into the old literature on instrumental and caesarean delivery it is replete with references to the *'rachitic dwarf'*.

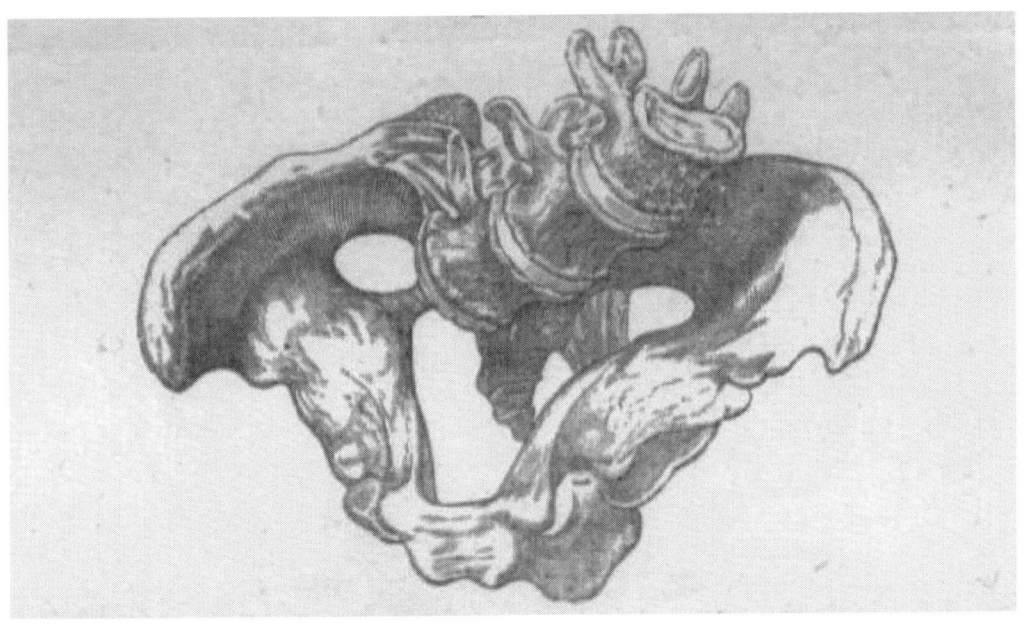

Figure 8.4
Rachitic contracted pelvis

Gebbie suggests that it was only in the 1600s that rickets became more than a sporadic problem, perhaps due to a change in child rearing: [36]

'Sometime in the seventeenth century, particularly in rural England, a change must have taken place in the rearing of young children. They must have been kept out of the sun and the open air and wrapped in swaddling clothes. Rickets would follow.'

Guilio Caesare Aranzi (1530-89), also know as Arantius, was a pupil of Vesalius, trained at Padua and became professor of Anatomy and Surgery at Bologna. His book of reproductive anatomy, *De Humano Foeto Liber* (1564), contained one of the earliest descriptions of pelvic contraction and the resultant obstructed labour. A translation of this was included by Eastman in his 1948 paper on pelvic mensuration.[38] Arantius outlined the type of pelvis that caused *'difficult labour'*:

'If, however the pubic bones, due to the fault of the formative faculty, have not been favourably arranged, that is to say if they are not too broad and in the exterior region so compressed that they become humped, rather than concave on the inside, and if they come very near the sacrum and coccyx, then the parts of the parturient become so narrow that the road is not wide enough for the fetus......"

He went on to describe the usual outcome of such cases: [38]

'And, what is worse, the helping hand of the operator which is about to bring aid, can not reach there because of the narrowness of the parts. Thus it usually happens that not only the fetus but the puerpera herself succumbs; sometimes also necessity herself compels the extraction of the child, which is already dead and putrescent, with difficulty and piece by piece.'

There are no details in this description to distinguish whether this pelvic contraction was due to rickets or to osteomalacia.[36]

Scipio Mercurio, whose text was discussed earlier, was a pupil of Arantius and therefore presumably familiar with his teaching on contracted pelvis. The harrowing description of contracted pelvis and its sequelae in Arantius's text may have influenced Mercurio's surgical approach to the problem.[36]

In the 17th and 18th century it was clear that in extreme cases of contracted pelvis the unfortunate woman was condemned to a protracted and painful death, as depicted in the following melancholy descriptions:

Percival Willoughby, who by all accounts was an estimable and compassionate accoucher, opposed caesarean section in the living, instead using internal version and breech extraction or embryotomy to overcome contracted pelvis and save the mother. However, in 1669 he was called to a case in which *'the pelvis was so straight and narrow that I could not enforce the instrument to take hold in any part of the child's head.....so I was necessitated to desist – not knowing which way to release her and she died.'* [17]

Pierre Dionis who, as we have seen, was opposed to caesarean section in the living recognised the link between rickets, contracted pelvis and obstructed labour: [19,36]

'But those who have had rickets when young are most of all to be pitied; for the basin in them is ordinarily so strait, that 'tis impossible for a child to get over the bar, or open a passage for itself. And now and then we see such women, after they have been in labour for several days, and have suffered most terrible pains, cannot bring forth but die at last.'

In addition to the above relatively passive acceptance of the woman's fate, an element of self interest was evident in some accoucheur's instructions – fearful lest they be blamed for the woman's death. Arantius discussed the difficulty of discerning *'the secrets of God's wisdom'* in these events and the potential risks to the accoucheur of using destructive instruments on the fetus with a moribund mother; resulting in his being blamed for the death of both fetus and mother. *'If however, the female parts, because of a relatively compressed pubic bone show considerable narrowness, I deem it better to take honorable flight and to withdraw from the task, than to take such grave hazards upon myself, the more so if the woman's constitution has been weak.'*[38] Scipione Mercurio expressed similar sentiments: [13]

'..... and also if she has a weak pulse, one must with justifiable excuses withdraw from the aforementioned undertaking; because, if perchance the parturient woman should die during operation, even though she should die from the pain endured, all the blame would fall on the operation and not on the other.'

Treatment options for contracted pelvis

Once a contracted pelvis always a contracted pelvis, and therefore the woman was condemned to the repeated horrors of labour and instrumental delivery – usually resulting in the death and dismemberment of her infant and not infrequently herself. Samuel Bard of New York recognised the dangers of being *'rickety during childhood'* and had sensible advice for mothers raising children about the value of *'exercise in the open air.....full but plain and simple diet.....walk, ride and dance.....and thereby fit them for safe and easy labours.'* [27]

The following options could be considered by the midwife or obstetrician –some in an attempt to produce a viable infant and others simply to sacrifice the baby to save the mother.
- **Induced abortion** was apparently used by the Greeks and Romans in women who were so deformed that vaginal delivery was impossible.[14] It was also carried out in Britain in the 18th and 19th century for women with a severely contracted pelvis and no hope of vaginal delivery.[21,34]
- **Restricted diet** during pregnancy was suggested in 1794 by a surgeon, Mr Lucas of Leeds.[39] The theory was that the growth of the fetus could be limited by a sparse maternal diet. This was not supported by clinical practice and was soon rejected.
- **Induction of premature labour** was first sanctioned in 1756 by a group *'of the most eminent men at that time in London, to consider the moral rectitude of, and advantages of which might be excepted from this practice.'*[24] The first case was undertaken with success by Dr George Macauley (1716-1766) in London. The procedure was performed using a quill or catheter with a sharp stylet to puncture the membranes through the cervix. This was done between the seventh and eighth month of pregnancy in an effort to achieve safe vaginal delivery of a smaller, but still viable child. It was applicable in cases of mildly contracted pelvis and was used with some success in Britain, but not adopted on the continent until the 19th century.[39]

- **Operative vaginal delivery** with internal version and breech extraction or high forceps could effect delivery in mild to moderate cases of pelvic contraction. This often resulted in a damaged or dead infant, but with survival of the mother. From 1890 to 1899 at Queen Charlotte's Hospital, London the perinatal loss was 77% in cases of internal podalic version and breech extraction done for contracted pelvis.[40]
- **Symphysiotomy / Pubiotomy** Operations to divide the symphysis pubis (symphysiotomy) or the pubic rami (pubiotomy) were introduced in the late 18th century.[16] For a time they were used in an attempt to enlarge the contracted pelvis sufficient to allow vaginal delivery – either spontaneous or with assistance of forceps or via craniotomy. However, the mortality was high and the orthopaedic and genito-urinary morbidity in survivors was severe and common. Furthermore, as it did not sufficiently increase the diameters of a rachitic pelvis, it was abandoned for this purpose.
- **Craniotomy / Embryotomy** were destructive operations designed to reduce the fetus into smaller portions and allow vaginal delivery to save the mother. Craniotomy involved perforating the fetal head, evacuating the brain and delivering the collapsed cranial bones. Embryotomy was the more general term used to describe the piecemeal destruction of the fetus. A number of special instruments were designed to achieve this. Most practitioners would withold this procedure until the fetus was dead, but if the mother's condition did not permit delay it had to be performed on the living child. These procedures were usually necessary with a severely contracted pelvis and were therefore very difficult for both the patient and the accoucheur. They could take many hours, even days, sometimes with breaks of several hours to allow rest for both parties. If she survived, the woman might suffer extensive trauma to the genital tract, bladder and rectum. For the accoucheur the physical effort could be extreme: La Motte declared *'the fatigue was so great that I was not well for several days.'*[41] The redoubtable William Smellie advised the accoucheur to pace himself for prolonged exertion, *' his hands will be cramped and enervated.....so that it may be a long time before he recovers use of them, and even then they will be so much weakened as to be scarce able to effect delivery.'* [42]

Early acceptance of caesarean delivery

With this background of reproductive carnage it was not surprising that some thoughtful obstetricians would give caesarean section another look. In this respect the French led the way in the 18th century.

It became apparent that with the severely contracted pelvis even the most skilled operator could not get access to deliver the fetus by craniotomy and embryotomy. In addition craniotomy was associated with maternal death rates up to 38%, and of course the fetal mortality was 100%. [8]

Guillaume La Motte (1665-1737) studied surgery and obstetrics at the Hôtel Dieu in Paris and set up as a surgeon accoucheur in Valognes, Normandy. He published his *'observations and reflexions'* after 50 years obstetric practice in 1721.[41] In the preface he challenged his teachers and spoke in favour of caesarean section in rare instances, *'.....if an ill confirmation was to hinder the introduction of my hand, I should make no difficulty to put it into practice.'* [41]

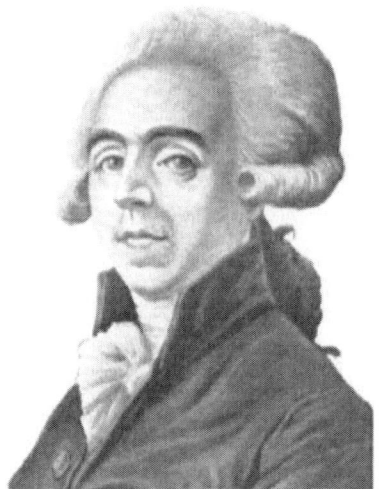

Figure 8.5
Jean-Louis Baudelocque (1746-1810. One of the early French advocates of caesarean section.

Jean-Louis Baudelocque (1746-1810) advocated caesarean section for contracted pelvis, saying *'with respect to the child, it is the gentlest and most certain of all the methods we can employ for terminating labour.'*[43] (Figure 8.5) He did however acknowledge the extra risk to the mother, and wrote *'But the mother having the same right to life, and this operation being generally fatal to her.....it ought not to be practised but when evidently necessary, and when delivery cannot be performed otherwise.'* [43]

Another early French proponent of caesarean section was Théodore-Etienne Lauverjat (d.1800), Professor of Midwifery at Paris. In his monograph on the subject he supported and performed caesarean section for contracted pelvis.[8]

Louis Velpeau (1795-1867) advised caesarean delivery *'when the smallest diameter of the pelvis is less than 15 lines (≈ 2 inches), be the fetus alive or dead, the operation of hysterotomy is the only chance of safety that we can propose to the woman.'* [44]

In Amsterdam, Hendrick van Roonhyse (1622-1672), known to his English colleagues as Henry Roundhouse, was one of the earliest proponents of caesarean section. In his *Medico-Chirurgical Observations* he wrote in favour of caesarean delivery *'.....when it happens that a woman great with child cannot be delivered, there should always a man-midwife be at hand, to save the fruit and to perform this noble operation.....'* [45]

The attitude towards the craniotomy versus caesarean section debate in Britain differed from France in part due to the Catholic Church's attitude toward craniotomy in the live fetus and the need for baptism. In addition, the experience with caesarean section in the British Isles up to 1800 was abysmal: 17/19 mothers died and 12/19 infants lost.[21] However, by the late 18th and early 19th century some British authorities acknowledged that caesarean section was indicated in the most extreme cases of pelvic contraction when embryotomy was impossible. It also became obvious that in such cases both the mother and the infant would die during failed attempts at delivery by embryotomy.

John Burton (1710-1771), who studied medicine in Leyden, Paris and Rheims set up practice in York, England. He advised caesarean section *'When both mother and fetus are alive, but no possibility of delivery in the natural way.....especially from the bad conformation of the parts of the mother, which will always prevent the operator's introducing his hand.'* [46]

William Smellie (1697-1763), the Scottish man-midwife who practiced in the slums of London and is regarded by many as the *'Master of British Midwifery'* [16] acknowledged the need and gave instruction for caesarean section[42]:

'When a woman cannot be delivered by any of the methods hitherto described and recommended in laborious and praeternatural labours, on account of the narrowness of the pelvis, into which it is sometimes impossible to introduce the hand..... in such emergencies, if the woman is strong, and of good habit of body, the caesarian operation is certainly advisable, and ought to be performed; because the mother and child have no other chance to be saved, and it is better to have recourse to an operation which hath sometimes succeeded, than leave them both to inevitable death.' [42]

Smellie did not perform a caesarean on a living women in his practice – always succeeding in achieving vaginal delivery via embryotomy if needed. He did carry out three postmortem caesarean sections for antepartum haemorrhage with no infant survivors.[42]

Thomas Denman (1733-1815), one of the leading obstetric teachers of London and known for his very conservative, non-interventionist obstetrics gave cautious endorsement to the early caesarean movement in Britain in the last edition of his book published in the year of his death[24]:

'Wherever it is proposed there shall be no other way or method by which the life, either of the mother or the child, can possible be preserved.....If such satisfaction could be given, I should consider this operation justified by every principle of religion, and the laws of civil society, upon as good and decisive authority as any other operation.'

Anti-caesarean school

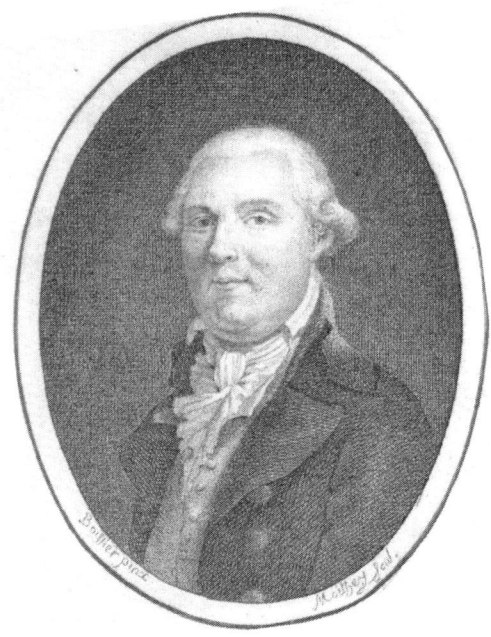

Figure 8.6. Jean-Francois Sacombe (1750-1822). Founded the 'Ecole Anti-Césarienne' in 1798 and called Baudelocque an 'assassin' for performing the caesarean operation

Jean-Francois Sacombe (1750-1822) studied midwifery in Montpellier and London before setting up as an accoucheur in Paris. (Figure 8.6) He was strongly opposed to any form of instrumental interference in childbirth – forceps, symphysiotomy and, particularly, caesarean section. He claimed that any woman could be delivered by natural means, especially in the hands of someone as skilled as himself.[8] He focused his most ferocious attention on those who advocated caesarean section – no matter the circumstances. In 1798 he founded and appointed himself leader of the *'Ecole Anti-Césarienne'* from which stage he lectured and published relentlessly against the caesarean operation: [8,47]

'This type of surgery is criminal and cannot be done because of the structure of the uterus as known from the experience of surgeons and obstetricians. The charlatans and liars who lead the pro-caesarean sects fabricate that such a procedure succeeded.'

Sacombe put forward his arguments in his obstetric text[48] and in a published didactic poem.[49] In his poem, *La Lucinade*, he claimed that while studying in London he was inspired by Lucina (Goddess of Childbirth) who appeared before him and commanded him to abolish the practice of caesarean section.[49,50] Short bursts of didactic poetry were not uncommon among physicians of the 18th century, in part to show their scholarly credentials – claiming that Apollo was the God of both verse and medicine.[50] Most medical didactic poems conformed to scientific accuracy but Sacombe degenerated into fantasy and slander.

Jean-Louis Baudelocque, a respected obstetrician and teacher in Paris, became the focus of Sacombe's vitriol. Baudelocque was an early advocate of caesarean section, albeit in highly selected cases where he deemed vaginal delivery impossible. After the death of one such case Sacombe called Baudelocque an 'assassin', both in lectures and in print. Baudelocque sued and won a high-profile court case in Paris. The fine was heavy, three thousand francs, which Sacombe could not pay. He fled the country, but returned in 1813 under the name of Laccombe. However, his practice was lost and he died discredited and poor.[8]

Opposition to caesarean section was not confined to the Ecole Anti Césarienne. In Britain the early results of caesarean delivery had been especially disheartening. Only one mother survived (in 1793) the first eighteen caesareans; the next maternal success did not come until 1834.[8] In 1798, William Simmons, surgeon at the Manchester Royal Infirmary, published *Reflections on the Propriety of Peforming the Caesarean Operation* and found absolutely no propriety in it at all, other than postmortem.[51] He accepted no indication for caesarean section in the living woman, regarding it as always fatal and dismissing reports of *'.....foreign accounts of success.....'*. He concluded: *'I hope that in the future all trace of the caesarean operation will be banished from professional books; for it can never be justifiable during the parent's life, and stands recorded only to disgrace the art.'* [51]

John Hull (1761-1843), a surgeon at the Manchester Lying-in Hospital, and the first in Britain to perform more than one caesarean section, joined the debate. The exchange became rancorous and inconclusive; Hull referred to Simmons' book as full of '.....*pernicious precepts, false assertions, garbled extracts, ribaldry, libel, hypocrisy, nonsense.*' [52] He pointed out that the caesarean operation offered at least some hope of maternal survival, in contrast to Simmons fatalistic view: '*Would it not be better that a woman die undelivered.....Life is in the hands of God!*' [51]

Thomas Radford summed up the situation: [34]

'*To my knowledge, there has been no subject connected with medicine which has created more bitterness of feeling and animosity in the minds of those who may be classed as Caesareanists and anti-Caesareanists.*'

Developments during the 19th century

A number of factors came together in the 19th century which improved the safety of the caesarean operation and changed the attitude of the medical profession. Most of these developments took place in the latter half of the 1800s.

- Anaesthesia (see chapter 13)
- Perioperative intravenous fluids, mostly saline, came into use in the 1880s.[53]
- The very high maternal mortality and the certain death of the fetus in attempted vaginal delivery with a severely contracted rachitic pelvis.
- Recognition that by delaying caesarean delivery until the woman was *in extremis* made subsequent maternal death a virtual self-fulfilling prophecy.
- Antisepsis and asepsis.
- Abhorrence at the performance of craniotomy/embryotomy on the live fetus.
- Extraperitoneal caesarean section (see chapter 10)
- Porro caesarean hysterectomy (see chapter 12)
- Suture closure of the uterine incision (see chapter 9).

Delay in operating

Robert Patterson Harris (1822-1899) was an obstetrician in Philadelphia, who had also studied in Paris. (Figure 8.7) He was an austere, temperate, bachelor who took a deep interest in obstetric statistics. His tenacity in tracking down cases made him the most accomplished obstetric statistician in the United States, and his publications received worldwide attention.

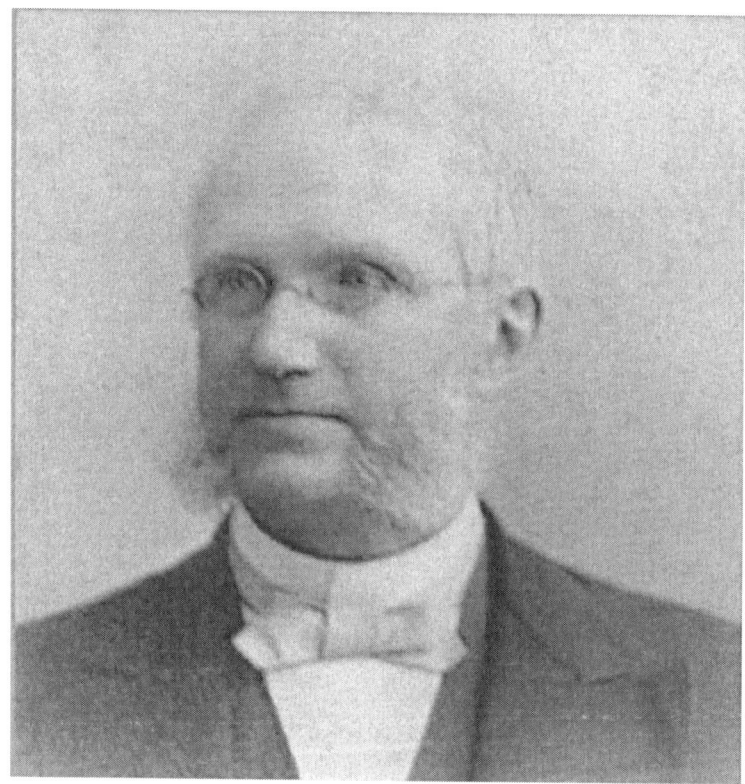

Figure 8.7
Robert Harris (1822-1899).
The greatest obstetric statistician of caesarean delivery in the United States; he advised its early performance in obstructed labour.

Harris was among the first to point out that delay in performing caesarean section, often associated with multiple consultations and pelvic examinations, along with failed attempts at vaginal delivery, almost inevitably led to maternal death:

'The accoucheurs consult, try various expedients, waste perhaps some more valuable time, and at last decide that there is no hope but in the caesarean operation, and the patient submits to the use of the knife to obtain rest from suffering, in a condition of exhaustion which is calculated to make it in a few

hours or days the rest of death. And then there is a grand hue and cry about the dreadful danger of the caesarean operation.....' [12]

It was, he argued, this delay and the resultant maternal exhaustion and infection that caused the mother's death, rather than the caesarean operation itself. Harris collected the first one hundred caesarean sections performed in the United States up to 1878, and compared the maternal and perinatal mortality between those who laboured less than twenty-four hours and those whose labour was more than twenty-four hours.[12] The results are shown below:

Labour	Less than 24 hours	Greater than 24 hours	Total
Maternal death	25%	66%	56%
Perinatal death	20%	77%	52%

These findings supported Harris' conclusion that the caesarean operation should be performed *'shortly before labour, or as soon as possible after it had begun'.* [54] He also pointed out that published case reports were biased toward successful outcomes. In the one hundred cases he collected the maternal mortality was 38% in published cases, and 68% in those he obtained by correspondence but not previously published.[12]

Thomas Radford (1793-1881), an obstetrician in Manchester, carried out a detailed and thoughtful review of the seventy-seven cases of caesarean section in Britain and Ireland up to 1880.[34] The maternal loss was 85.7% with the main cause of death attributed to an underlying *'.....progressive and incurable disease.'* Sepsis and haemorrhage almost invariably followed caesarean section, associated with prolonged obstructed labour, often with unsuccessful and traumatic attempts at vaginal delivery. Radford was one of the first English obstetricians to advocate early recourse to caesarean section: *'.....if the operation were earlier performed, and on a different class of subjects, it would be attended with infinitely more success.'*[34] The high maternal mortality in Britain compared to Continental Europe and the United States was notable. As Dewees wrote: [23]

'On the Continent of Europe, this operation is resorted to at an early period of the labour......The uterus is cut before it is inflamed, and the child is extracted before it has expired, and the attempts to save both mother and child is sometimes crowned with the happiest results.'

Harris, after detailed review of Radford's cases felt that the main differences, compared to the United States, were that in Britain: *'The caesarean operation being almost entirely confined to women of the lowest classes, who, by poverty of living have become the subjects of deformity of the pelvis.'* He also blamed *'Dampness of climate and extreme poverty'* among *'…..the beer-drinking female peasantry'* of England.[12]

Harris also pointed out that within the United States series only two of the one hundred cases took place in hospital; observing that the best results were obtained by *'frontier surgeons'* in remote areas of the country.[12,55] This he attributed, in part, to the lack of colleagues for consultation – which often added many hours delay combined with multiple pelvic examinations in the larger towns and cities.[12] The logical arguments of Harris, backed by his detailed analysis of cases in the United States and of the publications in Britain and Europe, were a significant factor in convincing obstetricians that earlier performance of the caesarean operation was essential for maternal survival.

In France, Cazeaux made a similar point, citing *'the almost constant failure of the operation in large cities, such as London and Paris, as compared with the success obtained in smaller localities…..'* [35]

Craniotomy versus caesarean section

If possible, craniotomy and embryotomy were used to deliver the fetus vaginally and save the mother the risks of caesarean section. This was universal practice if the fetus was dead, but much more controversial on the live fetus. The 1733 ruling by the Theological Faculty in Paris, that craniotomy/embryotomy on the live fetus was a mortal sin, had a strong influence in Catholic countries – especially in France. In the mid 19th century the incidence of craniotomy in Britain was 1 in 219 deliveries and in France, 1 in 1205.[8] Because of the high maternal death rate with the caesarean operation in Britain, craniotomy was resorted to unless the pelvic contraction was so severe than it was impossible.

There was much debate about the diameters of the pelvic brim, below which embryotomy and vaginal delivery was not feasible: ranging from antero-posterior 1½ to 2 inches (3.5-5cm), and 3 to 3½ inches (7.5-9cm) with the transverse diameter. Ramsbotham summed up the British attitude in 1851: *'Unless there be at the brim one and a half inches in the conjugate by three and a half inches in the iliac, it would be useless to attempt delivery by vias naturales.'* In such cases, he concluded, *'We ought to consider it a duty – however painful and appalling that may be – at once to propose the caesarean section as the only means by which it is possible to save the mother's life, and as offering also the sole chance of safety to the child.'* [39]

In 1859 Tyler Smith, physician-accoucher to St Mary's Hospital, London made a plea to abolish craniotomy and replace it with premature induction of labour, internal version and breech extraction or forceps.[56] He noted that craniotomy/embryotomy was carried out in about 1800 deliveries a year in England and Wales, or 1 in 340 labours. He acknowledged that '.....*cases will occasionally be met with in practice, in which perforation of a living child will not only be necessary, but a positive duty*'; but he described these as rare '.....*deplorable contingencies.*' [56]

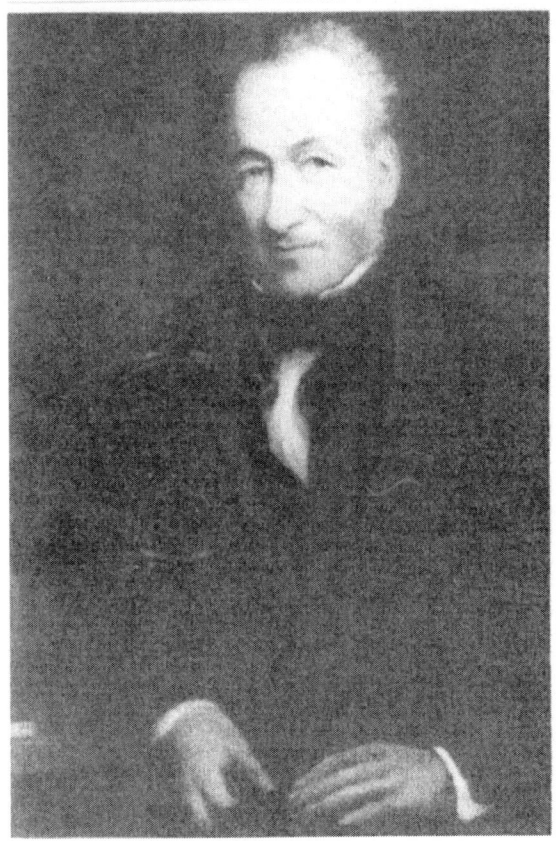

Figure 8.8
Thomas Radford (1793-1881).
The Manchester obstetrician was one of the first English proponents of caesarean section in place of craniotomy

Thomas Radford argued in favour of limiting the use of craniotomy on the live fetus (Figure 8.8.) He discussed the merits of the two lives at stake, pointing out that the woman's disease and deformity often gave her a very limited life expectancy. He declared, '*The infant's life ought not to be sacrificed for the mere ideal chance of prolonging her miserable existence, which is a positive evil to herself.*' [34]

Slowly, toward the end of the 19th century, the tide turned away from craniotomy in Britain as the outcome of caesarean section improved. Looking back on the era of craniotomy the London obstetrician, William

Playfair, wrote in 1876: [57]

'It must be admitted, however, that the frequency with which craniotomy has been performed in this country constitutes a great blot on British midwifery:......these figures indicate a destruction of foetal life which we cannot look back to without a shudder, and which, it is to be feared, justify the reproaches which our continental brethren have cast upon our practice.'

Caesarean section versus high forceps

One of the alternatives to caesarean section in cases of mild to moderate pelvic contraction was high forceps. It was recognised that the fetus could fare badly when delivered by high forceps but it would save the mother from the risks of caesarean section. Harold Williams of Boston collected a twenty year series of 244 cases to provide a comparison: 125 caesarean deliveries and 119 high forceps. The definition of high forceps was the fetal head above the pelvic brim.[58] The maternal death rate was: caesarean section 49%, and with high forceps 40%. However, for cases with labour less than twenty-four hours the figures were, caesarean 20%, high forceps 30%. As expected the perinatal death rate was higher for forceps delivery, 62% versus 18%. [58]

Antisepsis and asepsis

Much of the argument against the caesarean operation rested upon the seemingly inevitable post operative death due to sepsis; the cause of which was not understood until the middle of the 19th century. Louis Pasteur (1811-1895) of Paris and Robert Koch (1843-1910) of Berlin showed that fermentation and putrefaction were due to microorganisms and the *'germ theory'* of sepsis was established.[59] The English surgeon, Joseph Lister (1827-1912), used this knowledge to promote the principle of antiseptic surgery in 1867.[60] The idea was to kill all microbes in the surgical field with washings and sprays of dilute carbolic acid – which came to be called *'Listerism'*. This was gradually adopted for most surgical procedures, including caesarean section.

Up to this time, and indeed to the end of the 19th century, surgeons operated in their street clothes; at most they would deign to take off their jacket. (Figure 8.9). Rubber gloves were available from the 1840s, but tended to be used only at autopsies and anatomical dissection to protect the operator. For the same reason a few surgeons used them for protection in obviously septic surgical cases.

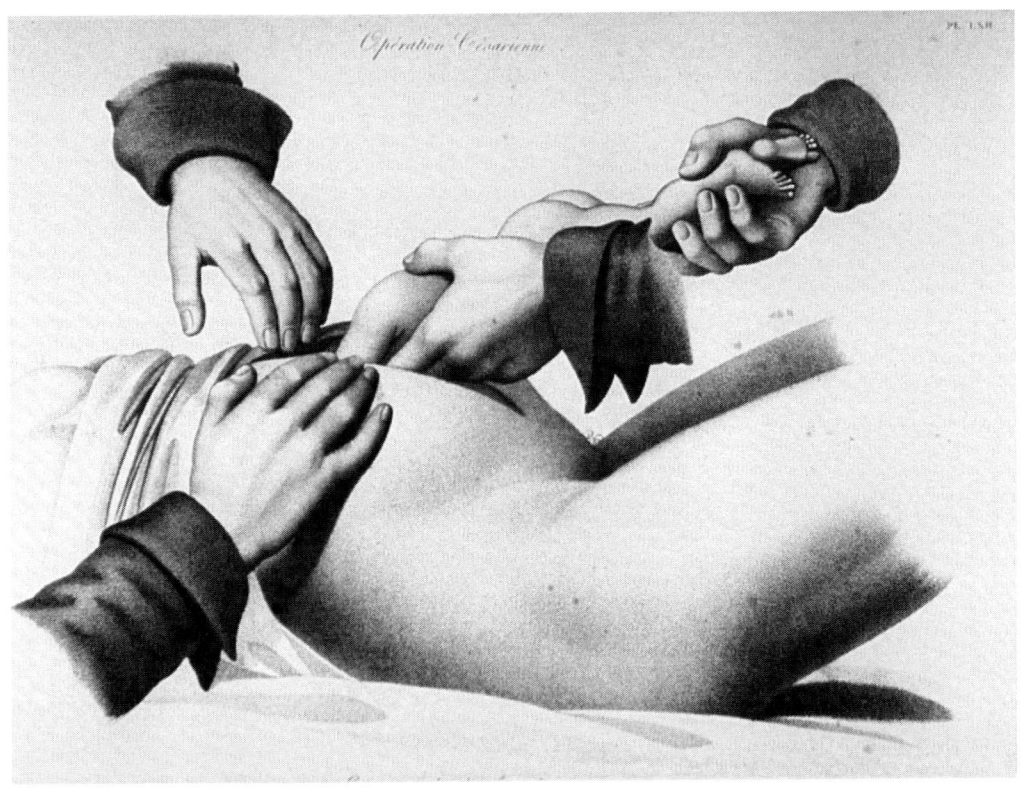

Figure 8.9
'Opération césarienne' before antisepsis and asepsis.
(From J.P. Maygrier, Midwifery Illustrated, 1836)

Surgical gloves only came into common use in the 1890s, popularised by William Halsted of Johns Hopkins University, because his head operating theatre nurse (later his wife) got dermatitis from carbolic acid washings.[59]

Some surgeons did not embrace antisepsis, but obtained favourable results with meticulous hand washing and cleansing of the surgical site and instruments. Steam sterilisation of surgical instruments, careful hand washing by the surgeon and all assistants, sterile gloves and surgical clothing comprised the basis of aseptic surgery. By the end of the 19th century asepsis (the elimination of bacteria) had replaced antisepsis.[59]

Early 20th century

The outlook for women undergoing caesarean delivery changed dramatically for the better after the 1880s, following the widespread adoption of uterine sutures (see chapter 9). In 1874 the maternal mortality in Britain, Europe and the United States averaged 54%, with a range of 33% to 87%. [61]

In Britain the maternal death rate fell from 27.7% in 1891-1895 to 8.1% in 1906-1910.[40] Amand Routh, obstetrician at Charing Cross Hospital in London, undertook a comprehensive review of 1282 caesarean sections performed in Britain from 1891 to 1910.[40] In cases of contracted pelvis, the additional risk of prolonged labour, particularly if associated with frequent pelvic examinations and failed attempts at vaginal delivery, is shown in the table below.[62]

Type / duration of labour	Maternal mortality
No labour or labour with intact membranes	2.9%
Labour with ruptured membranes	10.8%
Labour with frequent pelvic examination and / or attempted vaginal delivery	34.3%

In Britain and Ireland from 1911 to 1920 the maternal death rate was 1.6% for uncomplicated caesarean deliveries, but 27% for those with attempted vaginal delivery before the caesarean section.[63]

Therefore, even in the early 20th century, despite the greatly improved results with the classical technique, the fatal septic outcome in many cases with prolonged labour and vaginal manipulation was such that the obstetrician would still choose craniotomy/embryotomy if feasible, or the more radical Porro caesarean hysterectomy (see chapter 12) or extraperitoneal caesarean section (see chapter 10). However, for the period 1901-1906, Munro Kerr found a comparable maternal death rate for craniotomy (12.6%) to that associated with caesarean section (13.5%).[40] Thus for cases with mild to moderate pelvic contraction a trial of labour was undertaken, with an emphasis on limiting the amount of pelvic interference during labour. For a severely contracted pelvis caesarean section would be planned just before term or soon after labour started. The move to early or elective caesarean section was also supported by rejection of the long held belief – by then known to be incorrect – that well established labour was necessary for fully functional uterine contractility and the prevention of uterine haemorrhage at or after caesarean section.[55]

One of the earliest and most comprehensive population-based reviews of maternal mortality was undertaken in Philadelphia from 1931-1933 by Philip Williams (1884-1970), a Professor of Obstetrics at the University of Pennsylvania.[64] The incidence of caesarean delivery in the thirty-two hospitals with >500 deliveries per year was 2.6% (range 0.3% to 11.1%); for the city as a whole, including smaller hospitals and home deliveries, it was 1.8%. The maternal death rate among caesarean deliveries was 5.5%, of which almost two-thirds were deemed *'preventable'*. [64]

In round figures the maternal mortality fell from 60-90% before uterine suturing in the 1880s, to 25-30% in 1890, to 10-15% in 1900, to 3-8% in the 1920s. With the improved outcome came widening indications for caesarean delivery. The true conjugate diameter of the pelvis at which elective caesarean section should be performed was gradually increased from 5cm to 9cm by the early 20th century.[8] Cases of eclampsia unresponsive to other treatments and with an unfavourable cervix were considered for caesarean section. Placenta praevia was another condition associated with a high maternal and perinatal mortality and therefore potentially amenable to improved outcome with caesarean delivery. Before this, all cases of placenta praevia were delivered vaginally by some variant of *accouchement forcé* with internal version and breech extraction, cervical dilatation and lower uterine segment tamponade with bags filled with air or water, or by using the fetus as a tampon on the lower uterine segment and placenta via Braxton Hicks' bipolar version or Willet's scalp forceps.[16,65] In an 1888 review of the pre-caesarean treatment of placenta praevia, Charles Noble of Philadelphia reported a maternal death rate of 48% and a perinatal loss of 63% with accouchement forcé.[66] Noble was one of the early American proponents of caesarean section and he acknowledged the work and influence of Harris. Some idea of the gradual acceptance of caesarean section in the management of placenta praevia can be found in the different editions of the two standard obstetrical texts published throughout the 20th century: *William's Obstetrics* in the United States and *Munro Kerr's Operative Obstetrics* in Britain. In the first 1903 edition of *William's Obstetrics* he noted, *'it seems doubtful whether caesarean section will come into general use'* for placenta praevia.[65] By the sixth edition in 1930 he acknowledged that caesarean section had a place in selected cases. In the tenth edition, in 1950, caesarean section was widely recommended for all but the most minor degrees of placenta praevia. Similarly, on the other side of the Atlantic, Munro Kerr wrote against caesarean section for placenta praevia in the first, 1908 edition. By the fourth edition in 1937 selective use of caesarean was advised, and in the fifth edition in 1949 it was recommended that most cases should be delivered by caesarean section.[65] (See also chapter 16)

Caesarean section began to be considered for fetal reasons in the 1920s, as the maternal mortality in uncomplicated, uninfected cases fell below five per cent. The first reference to caesarean section for fetal indications in *William's Obstetrics* only came in the sixth (1930) edition.[67] Elis Essen-Möller (1870-1956) of Lund, Sweden posed the question in a paper on the role of caesarean section in 1924.[68] He asked *'Is it allowed to sacrifice the foetus only in order to lessen the risk of the mother? Is it allowed for the sake of the foetus to choose an interference that enhances to some extent the risk of the mother.'* In approaching this dilemma he quoted Theodore-Etienne Lauverjat, an early French proponent of caesarean section: *'The true obstetrician never sacrifices the mother for the infant nor the infant for the mother.'* [68] A noble sentiment, and one much easier to accomplish as the maternal risks of the operation fell in the 1930s and 1940s.

At the end of the 19th century the vast majority of caesarean operations were carried out for contracted pelvis or obstructive tumours of the lower genital tract. This was reflected in two personal series of caesarean section by Herbert Spencer of London and Edwin Craigin of New York in which contracted pelvis was the indication in 82% and 77% respectively. [69,70]

As the 20th century progressed the indications widened to include selected cases of placenta praevia, abruptio placentae, eclampsia and heart disease – albeit primarily for maternal rather than fetal benefit. The incidence of caesarean section as a proportion of all deliveries rose as its safety improved, although the national and regional variations were considerable – as they still are (table below):

Hospital / Region	Year	Incidence of Caesarean section(%)
New York Nursery & Child's Hospital [71]	1910 1927	0.2 2.5
New York Lying-in Hospital [71]	1928-31	4.9
Chicago Lying-in Hospital [70,71]	1915-16 1928-29	0.6 3.0
Rotunda Hospital, Dublin [70,71]	1920-22 1929-30	0.5 1.0
University College Hospital, London [69]	1920-22	0.6
National Hospital, Copenhagen [21]	1906-34 1935-45	0.4 0.8
Moscow [8]	1930	0.2
Norway [8]	1917-18	0.2
Denmark [72]	1941-45 1946-50	0.2 0.4

Already we see a tendency to higher caesarean section rates in the United States, and this would be sustained throughout the 20th and early 21st century.

The rising incidence of caesarean section in the early 20th century was not endorsed by all obstetricians:

Herbert Spencer of London wrote, *'Every thoughtful obstetrician must admit that caesarean section is being performed too frequently by certain operators both in this country and in America.'* [69]

Rudolph Holmes from Chicago was more forceful, *'Those who are now advocating caesarean section for placenta praevia, eclampsia and so forth must bear the culpability for the deaths which may result from uterine rupture at a later time…..but too often the obstetricians have wildly seized upon caesarean section as a ready and quick means of getting through with a case.'* [73]

John Whitridge Williams of Johns Hopkins University, wrote in the fifth edition of his influential text, *Obstetrics*, in 1924: *'At the present time I consider the operation is being abused and that not a few patients are sacrificed to the furor operativus of obstetricians and surgeons who are ignorant of the fundamental principles of the obstetric art.'* [74]

Andrew Hope Davidson, Master of the Rotunda Hospital in Dublin from 1933 to 1940, was so disturbed by the rise in the caesarean section rate to 1.3% in his own hospital that he declared: *'Some obstetricians regard the birth canal as a mere make-shift exit to be used only when they are otherwise engaged.'* [75]

The evolution of detailed surgical aspects of caesarean delivery are covered in chapters 9-12.

REFERENCES

1. Pickrell KL. An inquiry into the history of cesarean section. Bull Soc Med Hist 1935;4:414-53.
2. Rousset F. Traitte Nouveau de L'Hysterotomotokie ou Enfantement Caesarien. Paris: Denys du Val; 1581.
3. Cyr RM, Baskett TF. Caesarean Birth: The Work of François Rousset in Renaissance France. Cambridge: Cambridge University Press; 2010.
4. Sebezius M. German translation of Rousset's Hysterotomotokie. Strasbourg: B. Jobin; 1583.
5. Bauhin G. Francisci Rousseti. De Partu Caesaro tractatus. In: Gynaeciorum Sive de Mulierum Affectibus Commentarii. Basle: Conrad Vualdkirch; 1586.
6. Rousset F. Caesarei Partus Assertio Historiolog. Paris: Denys du Val; 1590.
7. Johnston TH. English translation of The Works of Ambroise Parey. London: T. Cotes and R. Young; 1634.
8. Young JH. Caesarean Section: The History and Development of the Operation from Earliest Times. London: HK Lewis; 1944. p22-92.
9. Pottiee-Sperry F. The hysterotomotokie or "Caesarean birth" of Francois Rousset (Paris 1581). The book of an imposter or that of a precursor? Hist Sci Med 1996;30:259-68.
10. Guillemeau J. L'Heureux Accouchement des Femmes. Paris: Abraham Picard; 1598. (Translated into English in 1612 by Thomas Hatfield as the Happy Delivery of Women. London;1612).
11. Rousset F. Dialogus Apologeticus Pro Caesareo. Paris: Denys du Val; 1590.
12. Harris RP. A study and analysis of one hundred caesarean operations performed in the United States during the present century and prior to the year 1878. Am J Med Sci 1879;77:43-65.
13. Mercurio S. La Commare O Riccoglitrice. Venice: Ciotti; 1596.
14. Graham H. Eternal Eve: The History of Gynaecology and Obstetrics. New York: Double Day & Company; 1951. p124, 164-70.
15. Raynaud T. De Ortu Infantium Contra Naturam Per Sectionem Caesarean. Lugdunum: Gabriel Boissat; 1637.
16. Baskett TF. On the Shoulder of Giants: Eponyms and Names in Obstetrics and Gynaecology. 2nd edition. Cambridge: Cambridge University Press; 2008.
17. Willoughby P. Observations in Midwifery, H. Blenkinsop, editor. Warwick: Shakespeare Printing Press; 1863.
18. Mauriceau F. The Diseases of Women with Child and in Child-bed. 2nd ed. English translation by Hugh Chamberlen. London: John Darby; 1683. p276-82.
19. Dionis P. A General Treatise of Midwifery. Faithfully translated from the French of Monsieur Dionis. London: A. Bell; 1720.
20. Ould F. A Treatise of Midwifery in Three Parts. Dublin: Nelson and Connor; 1742. pxxiii, 196-200.

21. Trolle D. The History of Caesarean Section. Copenhagen: C.A. Reitzel Booksellers; 1982. p37-42.
22. Lee R. Lectures on the Theory and Practice of Midwifery. Philadelphia: Barrington and Haswell; 1844.p311.
23. Dewees W. A Compendious System of Midwifery. Philadelphia: H.C. Carey and I. Lea; 1826.p578-90.
24. Denman T. An Introduction to the Practice of Midwifery. Volume 2. London: J. Johnson; 1798. p232-48.
25. Gifford W. Cases in Midwifery. London: Motte; 1734.
26. Chapman E. A Treatise on the Improvement of Midwifery. Chiefly with Regard to the Operation. 3rd edition. London: Brindley, Clarke and Corbett; 1759.
27. Bard S. Compendium of the Theory and Practice of Midwifery. New York: Collins and Perkins; 1807.
28. Speert H. Obstetrics and Gynecology in America: A History. Baltimore: Waverly Press Inc; p150.
29. Williams DI. The Obstetric Society of 1825. Med Hist 1998;42:235-45.
30. Transactions of the Obstetrical Society of London, 1859-1884.
31. Dunn R, Bailey HW. On the statistics of midwifery from the records of the private practice of Robert Dunn, FRCS and of HW. Bailey, FRCS. Trans Obs Soc Lond 1859;1:279-97.
32. Kayser C. De eventu sectionis Caesarean. Am J Med Sci 1844;7:489-92.
33. Kaufman MH. Caesarean operations performed in Edinburgh during the 18th century. Br J Obstet Gynaecol 1995;102:186-91.
34. Radford T. Observations on the Caesarean Section, Craniotomy and on Other Obstetric Operations. London: J&A Churchill; 1880.
35. Cazeaux P. A Theoretical and Practical Treatise on Midwifery. 6th edition. Translated by W.R. Bullock. Philadelphia: Lindsay and Blakiston; 1863. p842-3.
36. Gebbie DAM. Reproductive Anthropology – Descent Through Woman. Chichester: John Wiley and Sons; 1981.
37. Brock CH. The Correspondence of Dr William Hunter, 1740-1783. Volume 2. London: Pickering and Chatto; 2008. p184-5.
38. Eastman NJ. Pelvic mensuration: a study in the perpetuation of error. Obstet Gynecol Surv 1948;3:301-29.
39. Ramsbotham FH. The Principles and Practice of Obstetric Medicine and Surgery in Reference to the Process of Parturition. London: John Churchill; 1851. p311-22.
40. Routh A. On caesarean section in the United Kingdom. J Obstet Gynaecol Br Emp 1911;19:1-58.
41. La Motte GM. A General Treatise of Midwifery, 1721. Translated into English by Thomas Tomkyns. London: James Waugh; 1746.
42. Smellie W. A Treatise of the Theory and Practice of Midwifery. Volume 1. London: D. Wilson;1752. p341-91.
43. Baudelocque JL. A System of Midwifery. Volume 3. Translated from the

French by John Heath. London: J. Parkinson; 1790.
44. Velpeau AL. An Elementary Treatise of Midwifery. Translated from the French by CD Meigs. Philadelphia: John Rigg; 1831. p510.
45. Van Roonhuyse H. Medico-Chirurgical Observations. Englished out of Dutch (1662) by a careful hand, London: Moses Pitt;1676.p3.
46. Burton J. An Essay Towards a Complete New System of Midwifery, Theoretical and Practical. London: James Hodges; 1751.
47. Lurie S. The confrontation between the 'Pro-Cesareans' and the 'Anti-Cesareans' in eighteenth century France. Vesalius 2013;29:43-5.
48. Sacombe JF. Elemens de la Science des Accouchemens. Paris: Courcier; 1802.
49. Sacombe JF. La Lucinade. Poeme Didactique. Paris: Garnéry; 1792.
50. Marchal H. Poetic and medical codes in Jean-François Sacombe's obstetric epic, La Lucinade (1792-1815). In: Vasset, S (ed). Medicine and Narrative in the Eighteenth Century. Oxford: Voltaire Foundation; 2013. p211-28.
51. Simmons W. Reflections on the Propriety of Performing the Caesarean Operation. London: Vernor and Hood; 1798.p68.
52. Hull J. A Defence of the Caesarean Operation, with observations on Embryulcia, and the Section of the Symphysis, Addressed to Mr W. Simmons of Manchester. Manchester: R&W Dean;1798.
53. Baskett TF. William O'Shaughnessy, Thomas Latta and the origins of intravenous saline. Resuscitation 2002;55:231-4.
54. Harris RP. Abdominal and uterine tolerance in pregnant women, as shown by the low rate of mortality under severe lacerated and other wounds as the result of direct violence. NY Obstet Gynaecol 1894;93:111.
55. Eastman NJ. The role of frontier America in the development of cesarean section. Am J Obstet Gynecol 1932;24:919-29.
56. Smith WT. On the abolition of craniotomy from obstetric practice. Trans Obstet Soc Lond 1859;1:21-50.
57. Playfair WS. A Treatise on the Science and Practice of Midwifery. Volume 2. London: Smith, Elder and Co; 1876.p193.
58. Williams H. A comparison between the cesarean section and the high forceps operation. Am J Obstet Dis Women Child 1878;22:23-31.
59. Haeger K. The Illustrated History of Surgery. New York: Bell Publishing Company;1988.p206-16.
60. Lister J. On a new method of treating compound fractures, abscesses, etc. with observations on the condition of suppuration. Lancet 1867;1:326-9.
61. Charpentier A. Cyclopaedia of Obstetrics and Gynecology. Translated by E.H. Grandin. New York: William Wood & Company; 1887.p206.
62. Routh A. The indications for, and technique of, caesarean section and its alternatives, in women with contracted pelves, who have been long in labour and exposed to septic infection. J Obstet Gynaecol Br Emp 1911;19:235-52.
63. Holland E. Methods of performing caesarean section J Obstet Gynaecol Br Emp 1921;28:349-446.

64. Williams PF. Maternal Mortality in Philadelphia, 1931-1933. Philadelphia County Medical Society. 1934.p5,23,78-84.
65. Baskett TF. Of violent floodings in pregnancy: evolution of the management of placenta praevia. In: Sturdie D, Olah K, Keane D (eds). The Yearbook of Obstetrics and Gynaecology. London: RCOG Press; 2001.p1-14.
66. Noble CP. Treatment of placenta previa: a historical and critical sketch. Med Surg Rep 1888; 58:625-31
67. Williams JW. Obstetrics. 6th edition. New York: Appleton, Century, Crofts; 1930.p533.
68. Essen-Möller E. The place of caesarean section in the obstetrics. Acta Obstet Gynecol Scand 1924;2:244-79.
69. Spencer HR. Caesarean Section: With a Table of 120 cases. London: John Bale, Sons and Danielson Ltd; 1925.
70. Craigin EB. Obstetrics: A Practical Text-Book for Students and Practitioners. Philadelphia: Lea and Febiger; 1916.p790.
71. Hooker RS. Maternal Mortality in New York City: A Study of All Puerperal Deaths, 1930-1932. New York: Oxford University Press; 1933.
72. Shou P. The position of caesarean section in Denmark. Danish Med Bull 1954;1:29-37.
73. Holmes RW. Obstetrics, a lost art: a criticism of the promiscuous indications for caesarean section. Surg Gynecol Obstet 1915;21:636-43.
74. Williams JW. Obstetrics. 5th edition. New York: Appleton, Century, Crofts; 1924.
75. Gibson GB. Caesarean birth. Ulster Med J 1962;31:57-63.

Chapter 9

Evolution of the surgical technique of caesarean section

Preoperative considerations

The earliest texts emphasised the necessity of the surgeon seeking divine guidance; 'Having prayed to God, ...invoking God's help .....', and advised patients to '.....place their trust in God.'[1]

Consent to operate might be sought from the woman or, if she was *in extremis* when the caesarean was planned, from her husband and family. However, the surgical texts of the 17th and 18th century often did not mention consent at all, or did so in a perfunctory manner. Not so in the practice of Friedrich Osiander (1759-1822), Professor of Obstetrics in Gottingen, and one of the early proponents of caesarean section (see chapter 11). His advice to the patient about to undergo caesarean section two hundred years ago would comprehensively meet the most stringent modern criteria for informed consent.[2]

'It cannot be denied that of the women who undergo Caesarean Section more than two-thirds die, and barely a third are saved. Caesarean Section belongs to those operations of which the outcome is entirely uncertain. Before, then, undertaking this procedure, one should allow the patient to draw up her will and grant her time to prepare herself for death.'

Another 19th century obstetrician who emphasised informed consent was Thomas Radford of England, who, in 1880, wrote as follows:

'Every woman in whom there exists organic impediment to the passage of a mature or full-grown infant, ought to be at proper time informed of the nature and as to the degree of the obstruction .....if the cause of difficulty is great in degree, then the performance of the caesarean section will be required.'[3]

Before undertaking the usually mortal decision to perform caesarean section the early surgeons often availed themselves of consultation with colleagues. To some extent this was to share the blame for the almost inevitably fatal outcome of the operation. A typical case was reported in 1774 by the London surgeon, William Cooper, in which he consulted eleven colleagues over a twelve hour period before subjecting the patient to caesarean section; the mother died but the infant survived.[4] Harris pointed out that a prolonged consultation period was often the cause of further deterioration of the woman's condition and a contributing factor to the fatal outcome of many caesarean deliveries.[5]

By the latter half of the 19th century it was generally agreed that the main indication for caesarean section was a severely contracted pelvis such that '.....*a mutilated infant cannot possibly be drawn through.*'[3] It was further argued that most such women could be identified before labour (the ubiquitous rachitic dwarf) and that, '..... *since almost all patients requiring the caesarean section are in a wretchedly debilitated condition,*'[6] time should be spent in the last weeks of pregnancy trying to improve their general health.[3,6] The aim therefore was to make the caesarean operation an elective procedure rather than an emergency after a protracted, obstructed labour.[7]

Another consideration was the perceived advantages of awaiting spontaneous onset of labour and at once proceeding with the caesarean delivery. These advantages included maturity of the infant and improved contractility of the uterus, which was felt to provide better control of postpartum haemorrhage.[3,6]

For elective cases attention was paid to the site and circumstances around the operation. Playfair stated, '..... *it should never be done in a hospital, if other arrangements be practicable;*' and he recommended '..... *a large airy apartment .....*'[6] The operation was '..... *not to be made one of display ..... with very few persons present, and the greatest quietude should be offered to the patient*'; along with ' ..... *a genial warmth of atmosphere.*'[3] Cold air was generally thought to cause perioperative shock and many surgeons emphasised the need to warm the room. As Otto von Spiegelberg (1830-1881), Professor of Obstetrics at Breslau, put it: '.....*chilling of the open abdominal cavity is so dangerous; the temperature of the room ought to be from 22.5°-25°C.*'[8] John Aitken of Edinburgh sought to mitigate the effect of air on the peritoneal cavity by immersing the operative field in warm water.[7] However, there is no record of Aitken or anyone else putting his proposal into practice. Baudelocque advised that if there was time preoperatively '.....*it might be useful to prepare her by the general remedies, such as bleeding, purging, warm baths, etc as is done with respect to the other greater operations.*'[9]

The operation was performed on the bed or a table, preferably the former so the woman did not have to be moved after the operation. Most of the early surgeons placed the patient semi-reclining on cushions with her legs tied together and her arms and shoulders supported and, if necessary, restrained by two assistants.[7] From the earliest texts it was advised to empty the bowels (by enema) and the bladder (by catheter) before the operation. By the late 19th century Lister's principles of antisepsis were commonly applied with shaving of the external genitalia and antiseptic carbolic washes of the abdomen, and sometimes the vagina.

Abdominal incision

Throughout the era of caesarean section virtually no part of the abdominal wall has escaped the surgeon's exploratory knife. Rousset advised a longitudinal incision lateral to the rectus muscle – either on the left or right side, dependent on enlargement of the liver or spleen. The proposed site of the incision was to be marked with ink, across which transverse markings were made to guide the placement of abdominal skin sutures.[1] Oblique and transverse incisions – the latter was usually placed just below the rib cage to expose the fundus of the uterus, were also used in the 18th century. A number of the incisions were crescent shaped. The site of the surgical incision was often dictated by the area where the uterus most distended the abdominal wall. The early texts usually advised an incision lateral to the rectus muscle – mainly to avoid potential bladder trauma with the midline approach. This lateral placement probably accounted for the popular misconception that the baby was delivered from the mother's side or flank. By the late 18th century the midline incision became popular, with its advantage of speed and less bleeding. Fear of injury to the bladder dictated a higher placement, so one-third to one-half of the incision was above the umbilicus. By the mid 20th century the lower midline incision was in common use, to be supplanted in many hospitals by the Pfannenstiel incision in the 1960s and 1970s.

Most surgeons of the pre-anaesthetic era advised that an assistant should press on the sides of the uterus as it was being opened to bring the uterus forward against the abdominal wall and reduce the chance of extrusion of the intestines and to divert blood and amniotic fluid away from the peritoneal cavity. Others achieved this by having the assistant hook a finger in each end of the uterine incision and pull it forward in close apposition to the abdominal wall.[6] This was also done to exclude air from the peritoneal cavity, which many thought was the cause of peritonitis.

In contrast to the uterine incision, virtually all surgeons closed the abdominal wall incision with sutures, as opposed to bandages alone. However, drainage was, and remains, a very important surgical principle as Baudelocque emphasised in his late 18th century text: '…..*we ought to make two or three to unite the superior two thirds of the length of the wound. It is sufficient to preserve an opening of about two inches at the inferior part of it…..*'[9]

All surgeons bandaged the wound, and up to the 19th century compresses were applied – usually with a mixture of white of egg along with brandy or wine.

Uterine incision

Rousset's text advised as follows: *'The uterine incision is directed from top to bottom, between the side and the front, avoiding the site of the tubes and ovaries.'* [1] However, from the earliest times most surgeons made the more logical midline longitudinal incision in the anterior wall of the uterus. As caesarean section became more common there were attempts to refine and improve the technique. Different uterine incisions were tried to reduce haemorrhage, avoid leakage of the infected uterine contents into the peritoneal cavity and to improve long term scar integrity. These included both transverse and sagittal fundal incisions, diagonal across the anterior wall, lateral to the midline, and a gridiron approach with the outer layer of muscle cut transversely and the inner muscle longitudinally.[7] Even the posterior wall of the uterus did not elude the surgeons knife; although this entailed eventration of the whole uterus followed by a longitudinal incision in the posterior wall. The theoretical advantage put forward in 1881 by its proponent, Isidor Cohnheim (1841-1894) of Heidelberg, was that the weight of the uterus would compress the uterine wound and facilitate healing. Understandably this method, did not gain acceptance.[7]

The development of incisions in the lower uterine segment is covered in chapter 11.

Extraction of the fetus

Before the development of the lower uterine segment caesarean section the uterine incision was kept high in the body of the uterus, mainly to avoid potential trauma to the bladder. As a result the legs of the fetus would most often present at the uterine opening and delivery would be by breech extraction. The prize for the best description of this act must go to Jacques-Pierre Maygrier (1771-1835) of Paris: *'The operator then introduces one hand within the uterus, seeks for the child's feet, which he grasps and delivers with celerity and prudence.'* [10]

Occasionally the uterus would contract down on the fetus and trap the aftercoming fetal head. This was listed as a rare cause of perinatal death by Radford in his review of the seventy-seven cases of caesarean section carried out in Britain and Ireland up to 1880.[3]

'I mean the spasmodic seizure of the neck or body of the infant during its

extraction through the incised opening of the uterus. In such cases the body of the infant has been most easily brought along until the shoulder has passed, when the neck is instantly seized, and so firmly held, as to require long and continued efforts to be made in order to extricate the head.'

Playfair noted the same problem in his 1876 text: *'As the infant is being removed from the cavity of the uterus, the muscular parietes sometimes contract with great rapidity and force, so as to seize and retain some part of the body.'* [6]

This became less of a problem in the era of general anaesthesia for caesarean section, as this provided good uterine relaxation. However, with modern regional anaesthesia, which does not diminish uterine contractility, this problem has resurfaced at caesarean section for breech presentation. This is especially so with the aftercoming head of the preterm breech, which is relatively large compared to its body. Thus, it is now advised to have the tocolytic, nitroglycerine, available to give intravenously at all caesarean breech deliveries.[11]

Management of the placenta

In order to reduce haemorrhage and fetal asphyxia surgeons hoped to avoid the placenta as they opened the uterus. As Spiegelberg wrote, *'It is very unpleasant to meet with the placenta while making the incision, nor is it such a rare event, for that organ is frequently attached anteriorly.'* [8]

Radford went so far as to advise using a stethoscope preoperatively to identify the *'placental soufflet,'* and thus place the uterine incision to avoid the placental site.[3] If the placenta was encountered under the uterine incision it was either detached manually, if the edge was accessible, or cut through with the scalpel. When the placenta was not involved with the uterine incision it was either allowed to separate and delivered by uterine contraction or, more often, the surgeon did a manual removal. Some advised delivery of the placenta through the cervix and per vaginum to reduce further risk of wound infection.[7]

Prevention of atonic uterine haemorrhage

Until the advent of effective oxytocic drugs in the early 20th century uterine massage was the main technique used to combat haemorrhage associated with uterine atony. Baudelocque was the first of what was to become a long tradition of uterine masseurs, which continues to this day:

'If the uterus remains soft and inactive after the exit of the placenta we must touch it a little externally and stimulate it, to raise it from that state of

languor and oblige it to close itself.' [9]

Others put ice or vinegar into the uterine cavity or swabbed it with perchloride of iron.[7] From the late 19th century ergot came into use for this purpose.

Closure of uterine incision

The surgical texts from the 16th to the 18th centuries all advised against suture of the uterine wound. Leaving sutures in the abdominal cavity with its risk of sepsis caused by retention of this foreign material was against all surgical principles. Furthermore, sutures were felt to be unnecessary, as the following quotes from some of the early proponents of caesarean delivery show:

Francois Rousset: *'.....the wound retracts immediately after birth. This is sufficient to bring the edges so close to each other that no sutures are necessary and the wound seems to heal by primary intention.'* [1]

André Levret: *'.....not only prejudicial but absolutely useless because of the strong contractions which the uterine muscle undergoes after delivery.'* [12]

Jean-Louis Baudelocque: *'The wound in the uterus requires little attention: it contracts and diminishes more than half in a very few minutes. The reunion is the work of nature.....'* [9]

It would be some two hundred years after the earliest caesarean deliveries on live women before anyone had the audacity to suture the uterus. On 27th August 1769 Jean Lebas (1717-1797), a surgeon from Mouilleron in Western France, was consulted by a young colleague for a dead fetus with a shoulder presentation. Declaring vaginal delivery impossible, Lebas proceeded to caesarean section. He closed the uterine incision with three sutures (material not recorded) and also sutured the abdominal wound. The abdominal incision became inflamed but responded to wine vaginal douches and the woman completely recovered. Lebas did not report the case; but it was published by an observer, Normand Gallot, in the form of an open letter to a colleague.[13]

It was not until the 1880s, when the work of Kehrer and Sanger made a convincing case for careful suture of the uterine incision that it became the accepted technique (see later). In the intervening one hundred years only a few individuals reported suture of the uterine wound and this was often done out of desperation to control haemorrhage. Such a case was reported by James Barlow in England in 1817, although the patient died.[7] After Lebas the next two successful cases were by Weigel of Germany in 1838, and by Godfroy of France in 1840 – both using waxed silk stitches.[7] The first case of uterine suture in the United States was undertaken in Virginia by an unqualified '*charlatan*', observed by Weems in 1828 but not reported until 1836 after the operator had died.[14] Three uterine sutures were placed and the woman, after initially doing well, died on the 12th post operative day – reputedly due to the dietary indiscretion of taking meat with cider.[14]

The main arguments of the minority of surgeons who advocated suture closure of the uterine incision were: to manage bleeding, to avoid the egress of infected lochia and blood from the uterus to the peritoneal cavity and to prevent a loop of intestines from entering and becoming trapped in the uterine cavity. Others, such as Joseph Stolz of Strasbourg and Charles Rodenstein of New York, argued that the long term union of the uterine wound was jeopardised by its non-suture. They cited autopsy records to show that the edges of the unsutured uterine incision did not come together and heal, but remained apart and open. Stolz wrote: *'The uterine incision has no tendency to close itself, no matter how strongly the uterus contracts.'*[15]

On New Year's Day in 1871, Charles Rodenstein was assisting at a caesarean section and, after delivery of the baby, was asked by the senior surgeon to finish the operation. Faced with considerable bleeding from the uterine incision he instinctively closed it with silk sutures. Upon learning of this departure from surgical dogma the surgeon was so unhappy that, on the third postoperative day, he reopened the abdominal incision and removed the uterine sutures. Stimulated by this encounter Rodenstein undertook a review of the American literature on the topic. He collected more than four hundred caesarean sections done in 19th century America – with the remarkably good 43% maternal mortality rate for that era. In the fatal case reports he noted: *'In examining the post-mortem records, I am struck by the frequency of the expression the edges of the wound gaped, the uterine incision did not close…..I believe that caesarean mortality will be considerably reduced if sutures are used at all caesarean sections.'* [16] He was ahead of his time.

In 1852, Frank Polin of Springfield, Kentucky was the first American surgeon to close the uterine wound. He chose silver wire sutures which had been brought to prominence by the recent success of Marion Sims in closing vesico-vaginal fistulas with this material.[17,18] Between 1852 and 1880 American surgeons used uterine sutures in seventeen cases of caesarean section with a 43% maternal mortality rate.[16] The most commonly used suture was silver wire, with waxed silk, hemp and linen also chosen. Individual catgut sutures were found to be almost useless as, even with triple knots, they unraveled before wound healing.[7]

By the 1870s more surgeons in the United States, in Britain and on continental Europe were seeing benefits of uterine wound closure – particularly with silver wire sutures.[7] Harris, with his customary careful analysis of the available data was still undecided: *'Shall the uterine wound be left to nature or sewed up?.....The experience of our country is as yet entirely too limited to determine whether the employment of the uterine suture is, or is not, an improvement in the method of operating.'* [19] He later strongly endorsed uterine closure by suture.

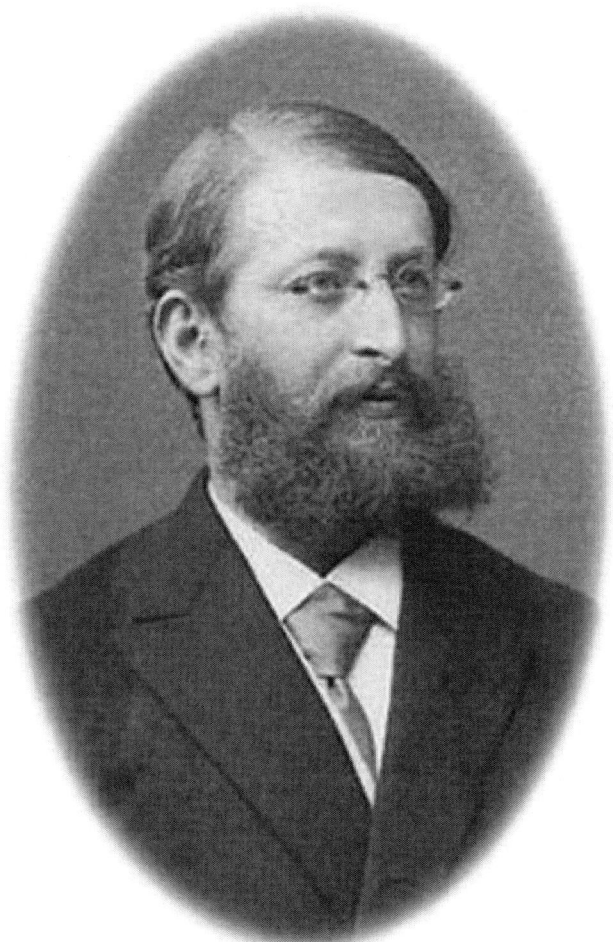

Figure 9.1
Max Sanger (1853-1903).
His detailed and sustained promotion of suture of the uterine incision led to its wide acceptance and revolutionised the safety of caesarean section

With this background Max Sanger (1853-1903) published his two hundred page monograph on the subject in early 1882 (Figure 9.1).[20] At that time Sanger was a twenty-eight year old assistant to Carl Credé (1819-1892), the Professor of Obstetrics at Leipzig.[21]

Sanger proposed his technique of uterine wound closure after careful observation, research and experimentation. As he put it: *'The salient consideration in the proposed improvement of the classical caesarean section is without doubt the treatment of the uterine wound'.*[20]

His work was not, however, based on operative experience. He acknowledged the published work of others – particularly that of Harris and the antisepsis principles of Lister. He advocated closure of the deep muscle layers with multiple sutures and ensured the close apposition of the peritoneal surfaces of the uterus by undermining the serosa on each side of the uterine incision and excising a thin strip of the underlying myometrium. In this way he ensured that the serosal surfaces on each side were coapted in a watertight fashion and without tension – the same principle as the Lembert suture for intestinal anastomosis. The deep sutures were of silver wire and the serosal layer was closed with individual silk stitches. (Figure 9.2)

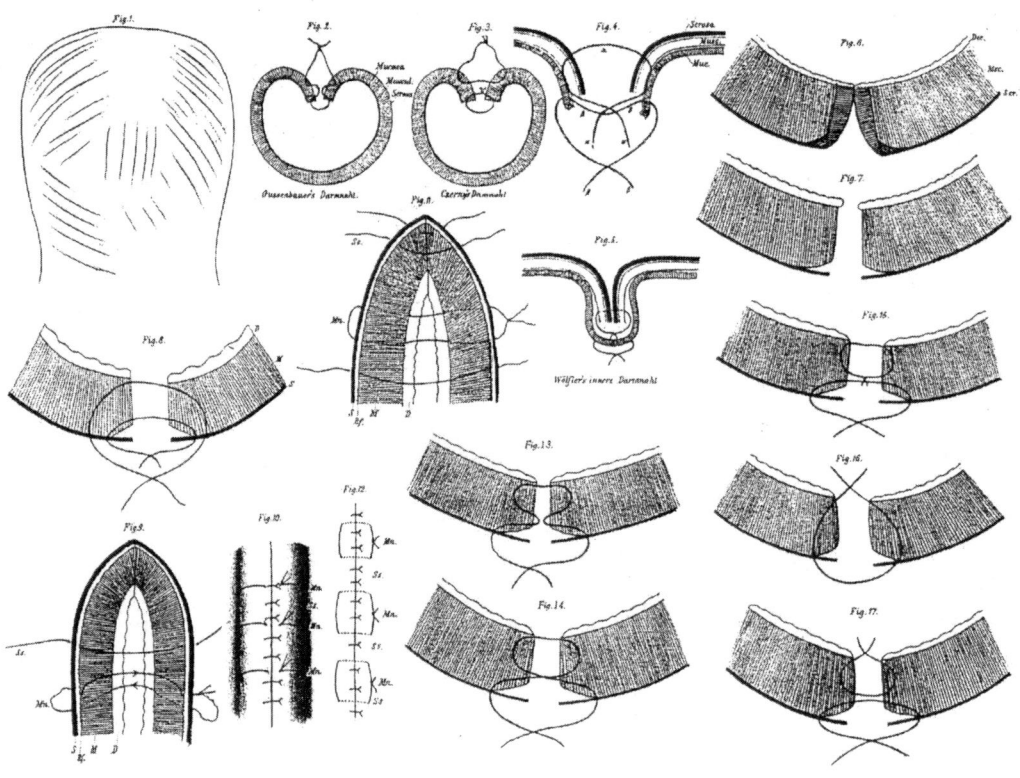

Figure 9.2
Details of suture techniques from Sanger's monograph (reference 20)

Christian Leopold (1846-1912), also an assistant to Credé, carried out the first caesarean section using Sanger's principles on 25th May 1882 – after the publication of Sanger's monograph. Sanger assisted at that operation, but did not himself perform a caesarean section using his own technique until 1884. By then Leopold had adapted the technique and omitted the rather bloody step of excising the strips of myometrium – a variation which Sanger endorsed. The procedure was dubbed the *'conservative'* caesarean section, in contrast to the more radical Porro operation (see chapter 12). It also became known as the *'Sanger operation'* which annoyed Henry Garrigues (1831-1913), a prominent New York obstetrician, sufficiently for him to publish an article on the topic in which he claimed to have performed a caesarean section using a similar technique, without being aware of Sanger's published work. Garrigues, a Danish – trained physician who had emigrated to the United States, wrote *'.....it may not be impertinent to ask, What is Sanger's method? .....Sanger has not even proposed anything new that in the hands of others has proved valuable..... there is little ground for attaching a single man's name to the operation in its present shape, which is the beautiful outgrowth of general surgical and special gynaecological development......'* [22].

Sanger was not at a loss for words when he defended his position with a letter to the editor that covered twenty-three pages of the journal.[23] He concluded his letter with an unequivocal salvo: *'Now that I have answered Garrigues quite thoroughly, I can calmly await the verdict of all impartial persons. I have the satisfaction of knowing that it will not be unfavourable to me, for right and truth are on my side.'* [23] Most people agreed with him.[7] At the end of the letter the editor of the journal declared the correspondence closed.[23]

Sanger also acknowledged the potential of the lower tranverse incision which Kehrer had used: *'.....the long cut in the middle third of the corpus uteri, the transverse cut in the lower uterine segment when there is an abnormal cervical dilatation, are methods that are most reliable and that should be tested further.'* [20]

Murdoch Cameron (1847-1930), of the Glasgow Maternity Hospital was one of the first in Britain to adopt the Sanger uterine suture technique, and did so with great success. (Figure 9.3) As a student he had been a surgical dresser to Joseph Lister, so he also applied Lister's principles of antisepsis. Cameron had the perfect population to benefit from safer caesarean delivery; impoverished industrial workers, with poor diet living in polluted, sun-deficient slums that led to a high number of rachitic dwarfs. (Figure 9.4)

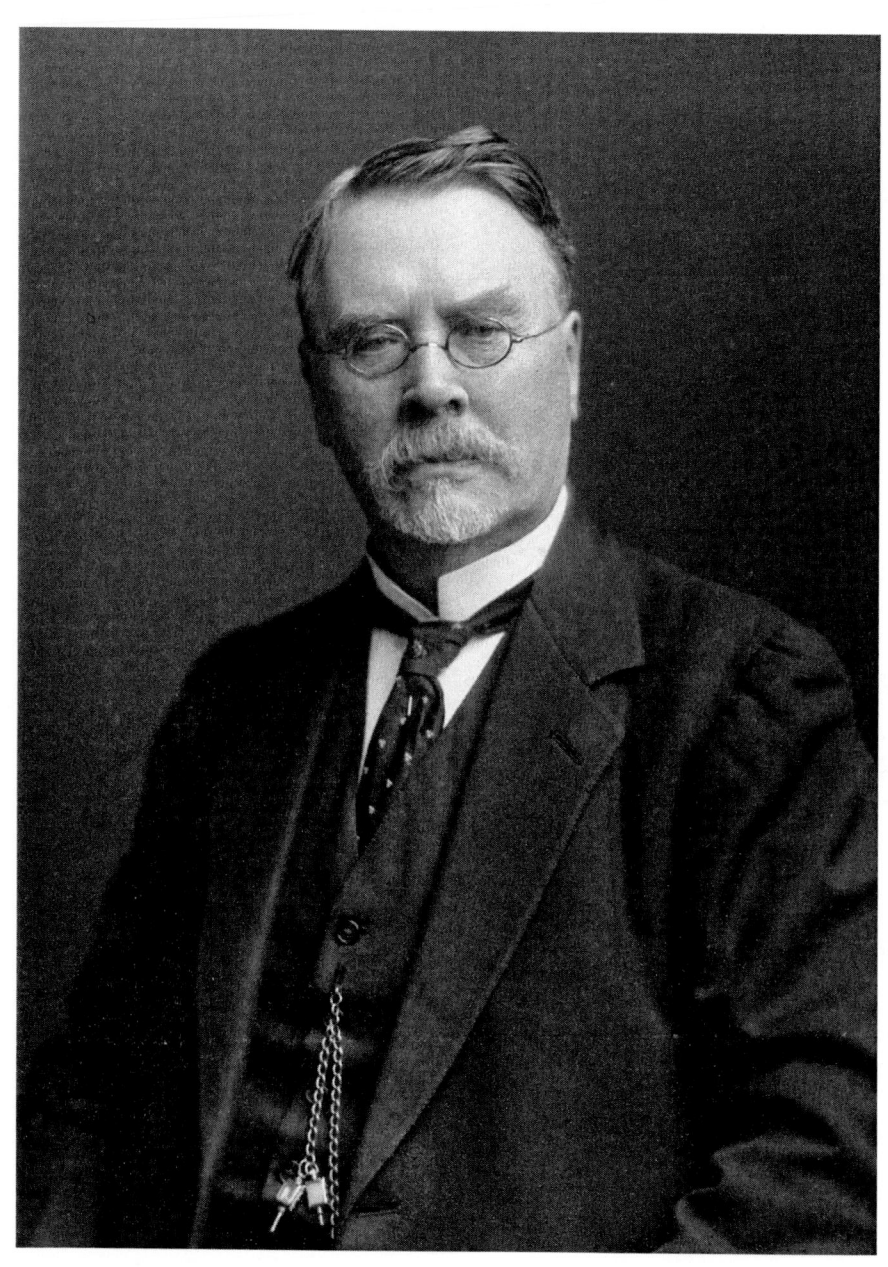

Figure 9.3
Murdoch Cameron (1847-1930)
In 1888 he adopted the classical caesarean technique, before or early in labour, in a series of rachitic women with such success that it became widely accepted in Britain.

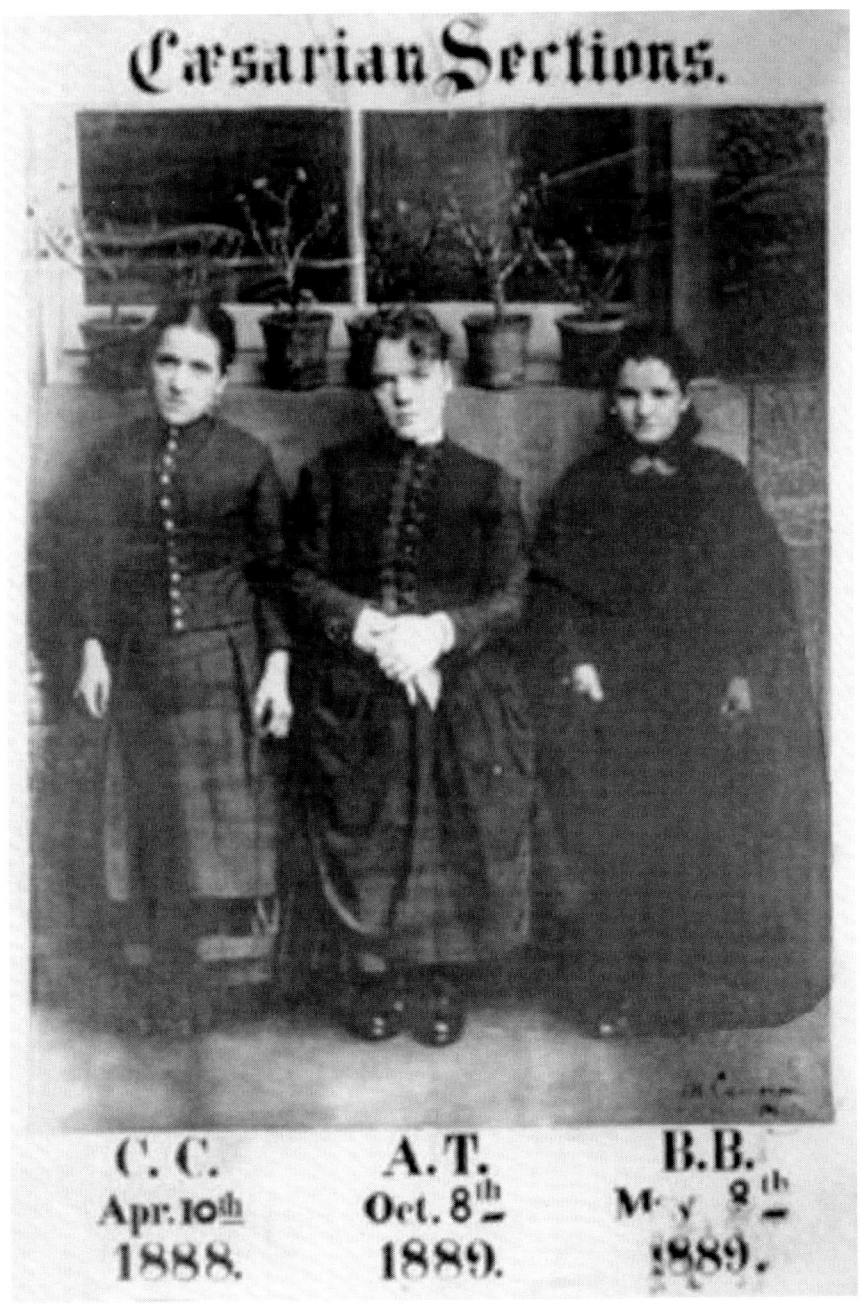

Figure 9.4
The first three cases operated on by Murdoch Cameron; the window-ledge in the photograph is about one metre high.

Between 1888 and 1891 he performed caesarean section electively or early in labour in twenty-three such women, with 100% infant survival and the loss of only one mother - an unheard of success rate at that time.[24,25] Reflecting on the alternative of craniotomy he wrote:

'I think the time has come when the lives of the mother and child may alike be saved, and I prefer to think that an infant, come to maturity, is destined for something greater than to have its glimmering life extinguished by an accoucher skilled in the use of a dreadful perforator' [7,26]

Of all the technical developments in the caesarean operation, suture of the uterine incision was to contribute most to its success and safety.

Sanger's principles of closure of the classical caesarean section incision remain in use, albeit with different absorbable suture material. The considerable contribution of Adolf Kehrer to uterine suture is covered in chapter 11.

Postoperative care

Rousset proposed two things to promote the flow of lochia and thus reduce the chance of sepsis:
- Long pessaries, made of hollowed out wax candles or cloth to reach through the cervix and facilitate drainage.
- Intrauterine douches with an infusion containing fourteen herbal ingredients including *'coarse red wine and good mead'* [1]

He also advised a diet of *'…..good meat and simple fare as much as her strength will allow.'* [1]

Scipione Mercurio also advised regular intrauterine douches, *'….to purge the matrix and to heal it and to strengthen it…..'* [27]. Other instructions included, *'….eschew the use of wine at least for a fortnight, lest it produce inflammation; and the woman must keep indoors, where air does not harm her….'* [27]

Baudelocque's advice reflected the 18th century obsession with bleeding and purging. *'If the woman is strong and robust, she may be bled some hours after the operation …..The belly must be kept open by glysters (enemas)…..a strict diet such as veal or chicken broth, very weak…..'* [9]. He also supported the rather radical advice of Monsieur Guenin, a surgeon of Valois, who, in the case of blocked drainage of lochia by blood clots in the uterus, reopened the abdominal incision, scooped out the clots and poured warm wine through the uterus and cervix to promote lochial flow.[9]

Nineteenth century surgeons all gave opium rectally or subcutaneous morphine for pain relief and catheterised the bladder every six to eight hours until *'spontaneous micturition'* occurred.[3,6,8] The emphasis on lochial drainage continued, and Spiegelberg advocated keeping *'…..the uterine cavity constantly irrigated during the first few days with …..a weak (1%) solution of carbolic.'* [8]

For postoperative bleeding Sanger advised wrapping the legs to cause *'autotransfusion'* and a *'salt infusion'* instead of early recourse to blood transfusion.[20]

REFERENCES

1. Cyr RM, Baskett TF. Caesarean Birth: the Work of Francois Rousset in Renaissance France. Cambridge: Cambridge University Press; 2010. p107-112.
2. Marshall CM. Caesarean Section: Lower Segment Operation. Bristol: John Wright & Sons Ltd; 1939.p1-31.
3. Radford T. Observations on the Caesarean Section, Craniotomy, and on Other Obstetric Operations. London: J&A Churchill; 1880. p24-32.
4. Brock CH(Ed). The Correspondence of Dr William Hunter, 1740-1783. Vol 2. London: Pickering and Chatto; 2008. p190-5.
5. Harris RP. Study and analysis of 100 cesarean operations performed in the United States. Am J Med Sci 1879; 77 : 43-65.
6. Playfair WS. A Treatise on the Science and Practice of Midwifery. Vol 2. London: Smith, Elder & Co; 1876. p220-1.
7. Young JH. Caesarean Section: the History and Development of the Operation from Earliest Times. London: HK Lewis & Co Ltd; 1944. p108-150.
8. Spiegelberg O. A Text Book of Midwifery. Translated from the Second German Edition by JB Hurry. Volume 1. London: The New Sydenham Society; 1887.p613-623.
9. Baudelocque JL. A System of Midwifery. Volume 3. Translated from the French by John Heath. London: J Parkinson; 1790.p356-7, 375-92.
10. Maygrier JP. Midwifery Illustrated. Translated by Sidney Doane. New York: Harper and Brothers;1836.p143.
11. Baskett TF. Essential Management of Obstetric Emergencies. 5th edition. Bristol: Clinical Press; 2015.p271-5.
12. Levret A. L'Art des Accouchements. Paris: Le Prieur; 1753.
13. Gallot M. Sur une opération Césarienne. J Med Chir Pharm 1770;34:177-186.
14. Weems ML. Case of caesarian section. Am J Med Sci 1836;18:257-8.
15. Stolz JA. De la suture élastique de l'uterus. Ann Gynec 1874;1:301-5.
16. Rodenstein CF. On the introduction of sutures into the uterus after caesarean section. Am J Obstet Dis Women Child 1871;3:577-82.
17. Speert H. Obstetrics and Gynecology in America: A History. Chicago: American College of Obstetricians and Gynecologists; 1980. p150-7.
18. Muffly TM, Tizzano AP, Walters MD. The history and evolution of sutures in pelvic surgery. J R Soc Med 2011;104:107-112.
19. Harris RP. The operation of gastrohysterotomy (true caesarean section), viewed in the light of American experience and success; with the history and results of sewing up the uterine wound; and a full tabular record of the caesarean operations performed in the United States, many of them not hitherto reported. Am J Med Sci 1878;75:313-42.

20. Sanger M. Der Kaiserschnitt bei Uterusfibromen nebst vergleichender Methodik der Sectio Caesarea und der Porro Operation. Leipzig: W. Engleman;1882.
21. Baskett TF. On the Shoulders of Giants: Eponyms and Names in Obstetrics and Gynaecology. 2nd edition. Cambridge: Cambridge University Press; 2008.
22. Garrigues HJ. The improved cesarean section. Am J Obstet Dis Women Child 1886;19:1009-10.
23. Sanger M. My work in reference to the cesarean operation: A word of protest in reply to Dr. Henry J. Garrigues. Am J Obstet Dis Women Child 1887;20:593-616.
24. Dow DA. The Rottenrow, the History of the Glasgow Royal Maternity Hospital 1834-1984. Lancaster: Parthenon Press; 1984.
25. Baskett TF, Calder AA, Arulkumaran S. Munro Kerr's Operative Obstetrics. 11th edition. Edinburgh: Elsevier; 2007.
26. Cameron M. On the relief of labour with impaction by abdominal section, as a substitute for the performance of craniotomy. BMJ 1891;1:509-13.
27. Mercurio S. La Commare O Riccoglitrice. Venice: Giotti;1596.

Chapter 10

Extraperitoneal caesarean section and peritoneal exclusion techniques

As already noted, during the 18th and early 19th centuries caesarean section was attended with a very high maternal death rate, and the majority of these deaths were due to septic peritonitis. Simple exposure of the peritoneal cavity to air was felt to be enough to cause peritonitis, while at caesarean section both air and the infected contents of the uterus were present. This chapter will cover extraperitoneal caesarean section and procedures aimed at blocking the peritoneal cavity from exposure to the uterine incision and its infected contents.

Extraperitoneal caesarean section

During labour and at full dilatation the cervix is incorporated into the lower uterine segment and retracted up to the level of the pelvic inlet. With obstructed labour the cervix can rise well above the pubic symphysis, as the vaginal fornices are pulled up and distended over the presenting part of the fetus. Most caesarean sections of this era were for prolonged, obstructed labour so access to the vaginal fornix via an abdominal, but extraperitoneal, incision became feasible.

The first to conceive and try this extraperitoneal approach, in an attempt to reduce the almost inevitable fatal septic results of the traditional transperitoneal route, was Ferdinand August von Ritgen (1787-1867), Professor of Surgery and Obstetrics at Giessen, Germany. (Figure 10.1)

He was probably stimulated by the success of surgeons who took the extraperitoneal approach to ligation of external iliac artery aneurysms. Ritgen attempted the operation, which he called *'Bauchscheidenschnitt'*, on 21st October 1821. The woman was in labour with a contracted pelvis due to osteomalacia that made vaginal delivery impossible; her general condition was poor, *'She was extremely emaciated, her pulse was small and rather rapid.....'* [1]

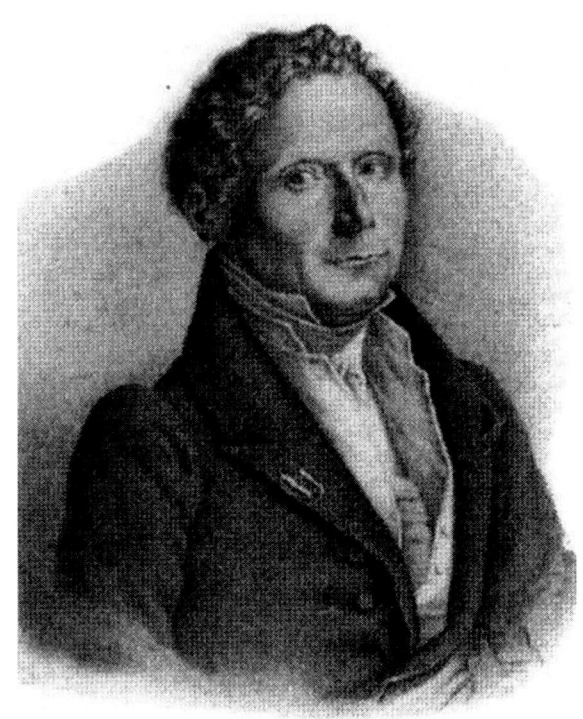

Figure 10.1
Ferdinand August von Ritgen (1787-1867)
The first to attempt extraperitoneal caesarean section in 1821

He made the abdominal incision on the right side from the symphysis pubis to the anterior iliac spine just above the inguinal ligament. Using a transvaginal wooden probe in the vaginal fornix he elevated this above the pubic bone on the right side and incised the vagina overlying the probe. Unfortunately, he encountered such haemorrhage that he had to perform an *'ordinary'* classical transperitoneal caesarean section to deliver the infant alive.[1] The mother died two days later. Louis August Baudelocque (1800-1864), a Parisian obstetrician and nephew of the more famous Jean-Louis Baudelocque (see chapter 9), attempted two similar operations in 1823, with the same fatal outcome in both cases.[2] Baudelocque called the operation *'gastro-elytrotomy'*.

A theoretical proposal for extraperitoneal caesarean section was put forward via letter, dated 28th September 1824, from WE Horner (1793-1853), Associate Professor of Anatomy at the University of Pennsylvania, to his friend and colleague, William P Dewees (1768-1841), Professor of Midwifery at the same university. In the letter Horner outlined discussions he had regarding the anatomical relationships of the peritoneum over the lower uterus, cervix and vagina with his colleague, Philip Syng

Physick (1768-1837), Professor of Surgery and Anatomy. He noted the loose cellular attachment of the peritoneum and its propensity to separate from the vagina, cervix and lower part of the uterus when the bladder was distended. Horner then outlined Physick's theoretical proposal to use this anatomical information as a basis for an extraperitoneal caesarean operation:[1]

'Dr. Physick, founding his ideas upon a similar observation made in early life, during the dissection of a pregnant woman, proposes that in the Caesarean operation a horizontal section be made of the parietes of the abdomen just above the pubes; and that the peritoneum be stripped from the upper fundus of the bladder by dissecting through the connecting cellular substance, which will bring the operation to that portion of the cervix uteri where the peritoneum goes to the bladder. The incision being continued through this portion of the uterus will open its cavity with sufficient freedom for the extraction of the foetus, all of which the doctor supposes may be done by a careful operation without cutting through the peritoneum.'

Horner knew that Dewees was preparing a second edition of his *Compendious System of Midwifery* and concluded his letter with these words: 'I have thought that even a proposition not yet confirmed by actual experience of its success would not be an unacceptable addition to the fund of information you are about to communicate to the public'.[1] Neither Dewees or Physick ever carried out the operation, but Dewees did include Horner's letter in his book.[3]

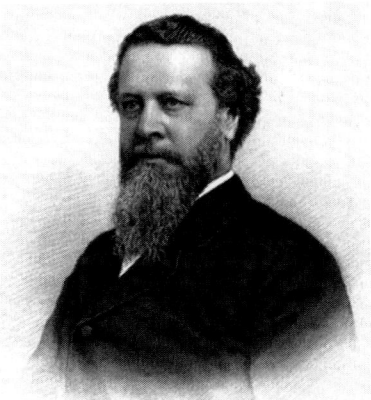

Figure 10.2   Theodore Gaillard Thomas (1831-1903)
Successfully revived extraperitoneal caesarean section in the 1870s.

It would be almost fifty years before Theodore Gaillard Thomas (1831-1903), Professor of Obstetrics at the College of Physicians and Surgeons of New York, revived the extraperitoneal operation in 1870. (Figure 10.2)

Thomas had practiced the operation on two non-pregnant cadavers and postmortem on a woman who had died undelivered of eclampsia. In March 1870 he carried out the operation, in a similar fashion to Ritgen, on a woman dying from pneumonia at thirty-four weeks gestation. The operation went smoothly, although the mother and infant died; but not, he felt, from operative complications.[4]

Thomas did not realise that his operation had been described before by Ritgen: *'I discovered that the idea was an old one and that which I had supposed originated with me, had years ago been tested and thrown aside'.*[2,4] Thomas performed his next case in 1878 with survival of both mother and infant. There were other individual cases in the United States and two unsuccessful operations in Britain. Alexander Skene (1837-1900), Professor of Diseases of Women at Long Island Hospital, Brooklyn, had the largest series with three successful outcomes in four cases.[5] Skene felt that the extraperitoneal approach was the best for infected cases. *'With each succeeding case I became more and more convinced of the great superiority of this operation over the caesarean section, for this class of cases. It is both easier and safer to do'.*[5] Skene called the operation 'laparo-elytrotomy'.

The Ritgen-Thomas operation had brief tenure for infected cases in the 1870s and 1880s. However, it was technically difficult, had a high maternal mortality of 50-60%, inadvertent opening of the peritoneum was common, as was bladder injury and subsequent fistulae.[6] Thus, at the end of the 19th century it was replaced by many surgeons with the Porro operation for infected cases (see chapter 12). Others continued with the extraperitoneal approach in an attempt to provide an alternative to Porro's more radical caesarean hysterectomy. The operative procedure put forward by Physick was, in essence, to strip the visceral peritoneal layer off the top of the bladder while keeping it intact. The bladder was then retracted downwards while the visceral peritoneum, now free of the bladder, was stripped off its loose attachment to the cervix and lower uterus – thereby providing extraperitoneal access to the lower uterine segment. This was easier said than done, and the few surgeons who attempted it soon gave up. The problem was that the space between the visceral peritoneum's attachment to the bladder was very thin and vascular, so that troublesome bleeding occurred and inadvertent opening of both the peritoneum and bladder was common.[6]

Wilhelm Latzko (1863-1945), of Vienna and later New York, simplified the approach to extraperitoneal caesarean section in his 1909 report of thirty cases with two maternal deaths.[7] (Figure 10.3)

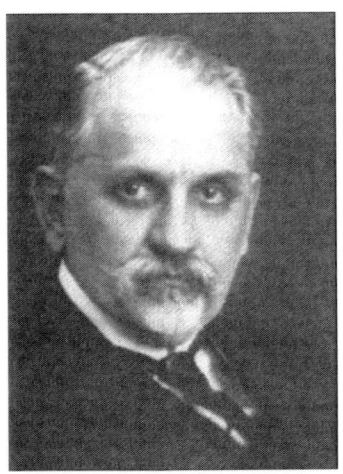

Figure 10.3
Wilhelm Latzko (1863-1945)
Introduced a simplified approach to extraperitoneal caesarean section in the early 20th century

Using a paramedian abdominal incision he opened the anterior rectus sheath and retracted the rectus muscle laterally. He then dissected the bladder and fold of utero-vesical peritoneum in the opposite direction past the midline to expose the lower uterine segment.

In Germany, Albert Döderlein (1860-1941) of Tübingen and Munich, and Otto Küstner (1848-1931) of Breslau, developed similar procedures.[1,2] In the United States, in the 1940s, Waters and Norton popularised modifications of the Latzko approach.[8,9]

Through the early part of the 20th century Latzko's operation, or modification thereof, was used when the extraperitoneal approach was advised for infected cases needing caesarean delivery. However, the procedure was more technically demanding of the surgeon, inadvertent opening of the peritoneum was common and serious bladder or ureteric injuries could occur. The operation was therefore mostly abandoned in favour of peritoneal exclusion techniques associated with the development of the lower segment caesarean section. The need for the procedure was also reduced by the availability of antibiotics. Interest in extraperitoneal caesarean section was briefly rekindled in the 1970s in the United States by a real or perceived rise in serious perioperative infection associated with caesarean delivery.[10]

Obstetricians experienced with caesarean section for obstructed labour in the second stage know how easy it is to mistake the stretched and elevated anterior vaginal fornix for the lower uterine segment. Robert Goodlin coined a modern name, *'anterior vaginotomy'* for this[11], and it is now regarded as a complication of caesarean section in such cases.[12]

Peritoneal exclusion techniques

These were not, strictly speaking, extraperitoneal but attempts to isolate the uterine incision from the peritoneal cavity by uniting the parietal and visceral (uterine) peritoneum or by suturing the parietal peritoneum directly to the uterus around the site of the proposed uterine opening. It was Kehrer and Sanger who, independently, started the principle of careful closure of the visceral peritoneum over the uterine muscle at the site of the incision; this has been detailed in chapters 9 and 11.

The first to deliberately try and exclude the site of the uterine incision from the rest of the peritoneal cavity was Fritz Frank in 1906; his efforts are outlined in chapter 11, as part of the development of the lower segment caesarean section. He transversely divided both the parietal and visceral peritoneal layers over the lower uterine segment and sutured them together.

Hugo Selheim (1871-1933) of Tübingen initially tried the extraperitoneal approach but settled on a modification of Frank's technique by suturing the transversely cut edge of the parietal peritoneum to the uterus above the proposed incision site.[13] For grossly infected cases Selheim felt this was inadequate protection and for these patients he created what he called a *'utero-abdominal fistula'* in 1908.[1,6,14] Using a vertical incision for all layers he sutured the parietal and visceral peritoneal layers and the edges of the uterine incision to the abdominal skin (Figure 10.4).

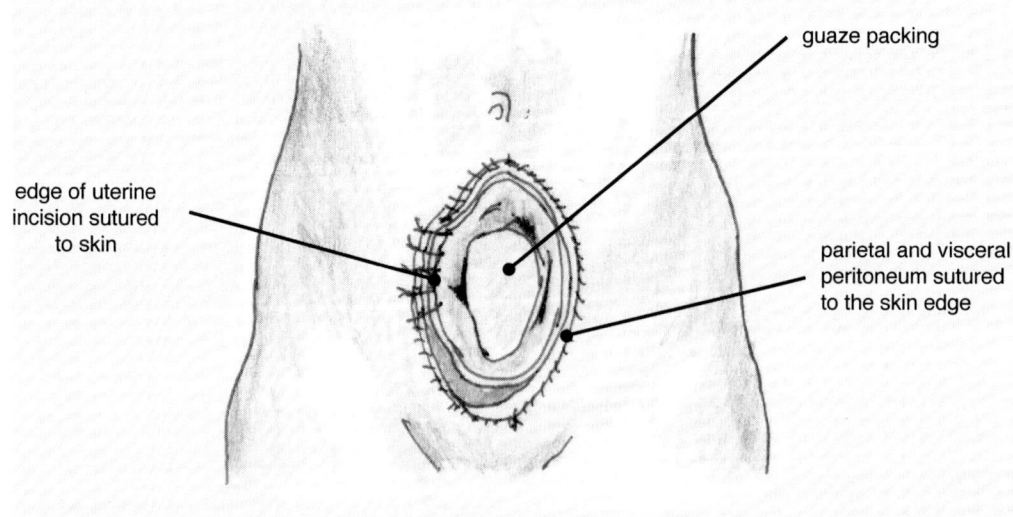

Figure 10.4
Selheim's utero-abdominal fistula, used in grossly infected cases.

If the wound did not heal spontaneously he closed it at a subsequent operation when all infection had subsided. In so doing Selheim was following the example of Pillore of Rouen in 1854 and Lestocquoy of Arras in 1857, who both used a similar procedure with infected classical caesarean incisions.[2,6] The same year, 1908, W. Rubeska proposed a similar operation for obviously infected cases. With a vertical incision he sutured the parietal to the visceral peritoneum, delivered the infant and left the wound open to drain.[2,6]

Johan Veit of Halle, Germany and his assistant F. Fromme reported a modification of Frank's method in 1907. With a longitudinal incision of all layers, they sutured the parietal and visceral peritoneum together and stitched them to the margins of the abdominal incision. After this exclusion manoeuvre they incised the uterus and, following delivery of the infant and closure of the uterus, reunited the two peritoneal layers separately and closed the abdominal incision. This became known as the Viet-Fromme operation and was used by others.[1,6]

McIntosh Marshall of Liverpool used a plastic sheet to isolate the lower uterine segment by suturing the edges of a slit in the plastic to the utero-vesical peritoneum.[1]

Other methods to decrease the risks of peritonitis

It is appropriate here to review the other methods used to reduce the risks of infection in potentially or obviously infected women coming to caesarean section:
- In the early 20th century some obstetricians still advocated delivering the placenta through the cervix and vagina after caesarean section, despite the fact that the infant had already been delivered through the uterine wound. Once such advocate was Munro Kerr.[15]
- Avoidance of the Trendelenburg position in favour of the horizontal to avoid spill of the uterine contents to the upper peritoneal cavity at the time of uterine incision.
- Careful packing with gauze of the peritoneal pouches at the side of the uterus to collect any uterine spill.
- Aspiration of the amniotic fluid via catheter through a small initial uterine incision. This could lead to fetal asphyxia and was never shown to be of benefit.[1]
- Eventration of the uterus and careful packing around the abdominal wound before making the uterine incision. This technique was favoured by Heinrich Doerfler in Germany, but required a very large incision.[1]

Portes operation

This two-stage procedure was developed in 1923 by Louis Portes (1891-1850) of Paris for use in neglected cases with advanced sepsis that required caesarean delivery.[16] In the first stage the uterus was delivered through a large longitudinal abdominal incision which was then closed behind the uterus down to the cervix. The fetus and placenta were then delivered through a high vertical uterine incision. The uterine incision was sutured and the uterus left to involute on the outside of the abdominal wall. Provided the sepsis subsided the abdomen was reopened three to eight weeks later, the uterus and adnexa returned to the pelvic cavity and the abdominal wall closed. If the sepsis continued, hysterectomy of the exteriorised uterus was carried out. To a limited degree this operation found favour, mainly in France, for cases of advanced sepsis and as an alternative to Porro's operation allowing, as it did, a chance of uterine preservation.[2,17]

Vaginal caesarean section

This was developed by Alfred Duhrssen (1862-1933), Professor of Obstetrics in Berlin. His first approach, in 1890, was to remove the obstruction to vaginal delivery of an incompletely dilated cervix in labour by four cervical incisions: two lateral, one anterior and one posterior. These came to be called Duhrssen's incisions.[18]

He extended this principle to the more radical vaginal caesarean section for rare cases in which rapid delivery was necessary – some cases of eclampsia, placenta praevia, cord prolapse and maternal death with a live fetus. The advantage, he claimed, compared to abdominal caesarean section, was speed and less maternal morbidity than with an abdominal incision entering the peritoneal cavity.[19] The technique involved incising the skin over the anterior and posterior cervix to allow dissection of the bladder and pouch of Douglas peritoneal sac upwards. The body of the cervix was then cut front and back up to the lower uterine segment, allowing access to the fetal presenting part which could then be delivered by forceps or breech extraction. Sometimes only the anterior incision was necessary.[20]

Many, including Munro Kerr, felt the technique had a place when termination was necessary in the first half of pregnancy, but few thought it appropriate for a viable term fetus.[21] Routh reported forty-three cases in Britain between 1895 and 1910, mostly in the early months of pregnancy, with a maternal mortality of 32.6%.[22] It had brief currency with some obstetricians, mostly in Germany, but as abdominal caesarean section became safer it was abandoned.

REFERENCES

1. Marshall CM. Caesarean Section: Lower Segment Operation. Bristol: John Wright & Sons Ltd; 1939. p1-31.
2. Young JH. Caesarean Section: The History and Development of the Operation from Earliest Times. London: HK Lewis & Co Ltd; 1944. p190-223.
3. Dewees WP. A Compendious System of Midwifery. 2nd edition. Philadelphia: H.C. Carey & I. Lea; 1826. p590-2.
4. Thomas TG. Gastro-elytrotomy: a substitute for caesarean section. Am J Obstet Dis Woman Child 1871;3:125-39.
5. Skene AJC. A successful case of laparo-elytrotomy with remarks on the operation. Ann Surg 1885;1:25-9.
6. Ricci JV, Marr JP. Principles of Extraperitoneal Caesarean Section. Philadelphia: The Blakiston Company; 1942.
7. Latzko W. Uber den extraperitonealen Kaiserschnitt. Zentralbl Gynakol 1909;33:275-82.
8. Waters EG. Supravesical extraperitoneal cesarean section: presentation of a new technic. Am J Obstet Gynecol 1940;39:423-8.
9. Norton JF. A paravesical extraperitoneal cesarean section technique. Am J Obstet Gynecol 1946;51:519-24.
10. Imig JR, Perkins RP. Extraperitoneal cesarean section. A new need for old skills. Am J Obstet Gynecol 1976;125:51-7.
11. Goodlin RC. Anterior vaginotomy: abdominal delivery without a uterine incision. Obstet Gynecol 1996;88:467-9.
12. Gortzak-Uzan L, Walfisch A, Gortzak Y, Katz M, Mazor M, Hallak M. Accidental vaginal incision during cesarean section: a report of four cases. J Reprod Med 2001;46:101720.
13. Selheim H. Der extraperitonealen uterusschnitt. Zentralbl Gynakol. 1908;32:133-42.
14. Wilson JR. The conquest of cesarean section-related infections: progress report. Obstet Gynecol 1988;72:519-32.
15. Kerr JM. Operative Midwifery. 2nd edition. London: Balliere, Tindall and Cox; 1911. p416.
16. Portes L. La césarienne suivie d'extériorisation de l'utérus. Gynec Obstet 1924;10:225-32.
17. Phaneuf LE. Caesarean section followed by temporary exteriorisation of the uterus: The Portes Operation. Surg Gynecol Obstet 1927;44:788-94.
18. Baskett T.F. On the Shoulders of Giants: Eponyms and Names in Obstetrics and Gynaecology. Cambridge: Cambridge University Press;2008.p110-11.

19. Duhrssen A. Ein neuer Fall von vaginalen Kaiserschnitt. Arch Gynakol. 1896;61:548-64.
20. Davis EP. Operative Obstetrics. Philadelphia: WB Saunders Company;1911; p289-99.
21. Kerr JM. Operative Midwifery. London: Balliere, Tindall and Cox;1908. p469-77.
22. Routh A. On caesarean section in the United Kingdom. J Obstet Gynaecol Br Emp 1911;19:1-58.

Chapter 11

Lower uterine segment caesarean section

In 1786 Robert Wallace Johnson, the London obstetric surgeon and former pupil of William Smellie, was the first to suggest that the uterine incision for caesarean section might best be made in the lower part of the uterus. He based his opinion on the review of two cases of uterine rupture in labour reported by colleagues.[1,2] Both ruptures occurred during the second stage of labour, involved the uterus just above the cervix and, after vaginal delivery of the infant, there was very little bleeding and the women recovered. Johnson extrapolated this outcome to the almost universal fatal results of caesarean section at that time and proposed the following approach to the operation:

'I would have the incision made through the uterus transversely on its anterior side, as near the cervix as not to injure the bladder; avoiding as much as possible the larger branches of the hypogastric arteries; and this aperture being made of sufficient largeness, then to pass the end of a male catheter through a puncture made in the membranes to draw off the liquor amni etc, so then an effusion thereof may not gush into the general cavity of the abdomen. If these few particulars are adopted .....I should hope that better success would attend hysterotomy.'[1,2]

It was to be almost one hundred years before Kehrer adopted this principle and a further fifty years before Kehrer's technique, which was essentially the modern lower segment caesarean procedure, was widely accepted.[3] The intervening one hundred and fifty years form the background of this chapter.

The 19th century was an era of considerable innovation in German surgery, particularly in the specialty of obstetrics and gynaecology. One such innovator was Friedrich Benjamin Osiander (1759-1822), Professor of Obstetrics in Gottingen from 1792 until his death in 1822. (Figure 11.1) Confronting the high mortality due to haemorrhage and sepsis associated with the classical upper uterine segment caesarean, Osiander sought another route:

'There still remains another type of incision, devised by myself, which opens the uterus in its lower half, and through which, with less danger, the delivery of the child may quickly be brought about.'[4,5]

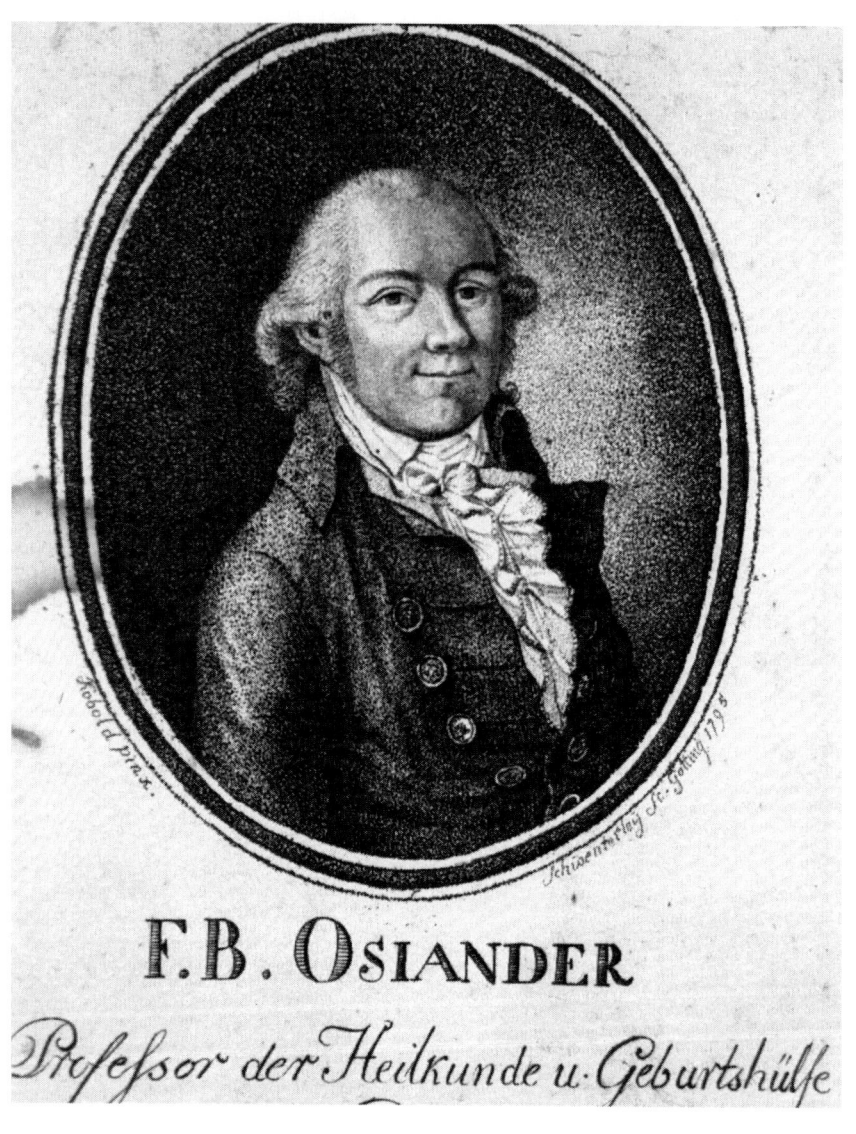

Figure 11.1
Friedrich Benjamin Osiander (1759-1822)

He outlined the advantages of using the lower part of the uterus as, (a) needing a smaller uterine incision, (b) the uterine wound lay behind the symphysis and therefore entrapment of bowel was unlikely and, (c) the sequelae of rupture of the lower uterus were less than that of the upper uterine segment – as Johnson had previously noticed. It was Osiander's predecessor in Gottingen, Johan Georg Roederer (1727-1763), who first used the term 'lower uterine segment'.[6]

Osiander's first case was performed on 20th March, 1805 on the proverbial rachitic dwarf, whose general medical condition was described as *'pitiable'*. Her contracted pelvis precluded all attempts at vaginal delivery. Seated between the patient's legs Osiander placed his left hand into the vagina and pushed the fetal head against the lower abdominal wall. With his right hand he made a vertical incision over the fetal head and *'exposed the uterus at the third stroke.'* [4,5] He continued the vertical incision through the uterus and pushed the fetal head through the uterine opening (Figure 11.2). The infant and placenta were delivered with ease. Osiander noted very little uterine bleeding, did not suture the uterus, but did close the abdomen with four stitches. The patient died a few hours later.[4,5]

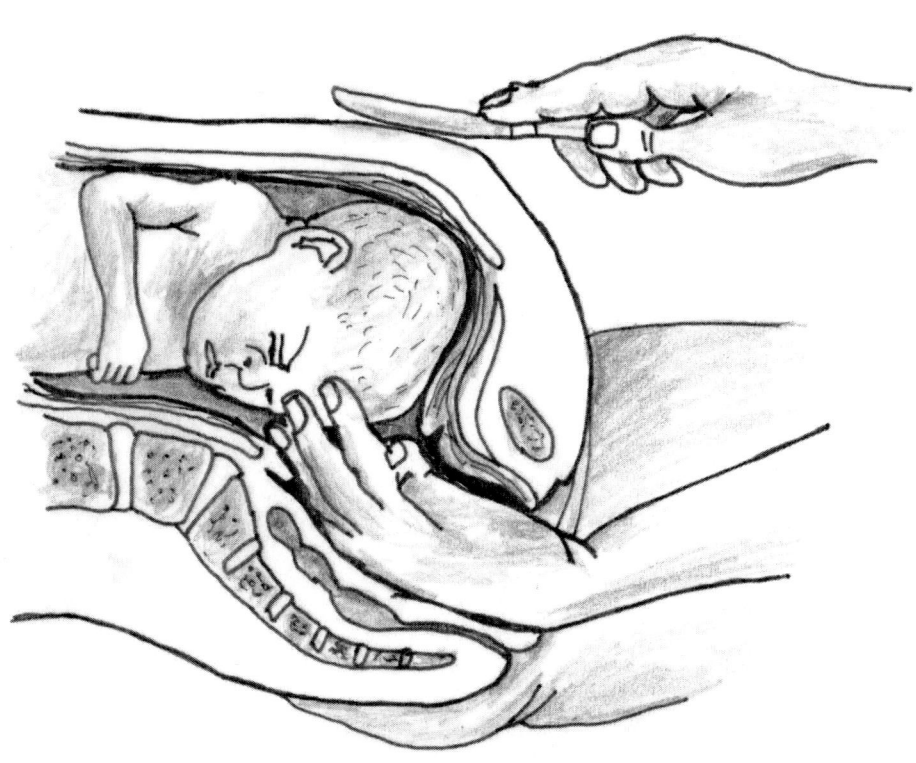

Figure 11.2
Osiander's lower uterine segment operation

Another German obstetrician, Johan Jörg of Leipzig (1779-1856), came to a similar conclusion on theoretical grounds in 1806:

'The vagina is occasionally ruptured in difficult and tedious labours, and the child generally escapes through the tear into the peritoneal cavity .....Would it not be possible in performing Caesarean section to open the vagina, and, where this is not sufficient, to extend the incision into the uterus?' [5]

Jörg never performed this type of caesarean section, except once on a cadaver. Whether he came to his conclusion independently or was aware of Osiander's work, at that time unpublished, is moot. Both Osiander and Jörg's methods involved opening the peritoneal cavity with its attendant risks of an often fatal septic outcome. For much of the 19th century, therefore, attempts to perfect extraperitoneal caesarean techniques were pursued (see chapter 10).

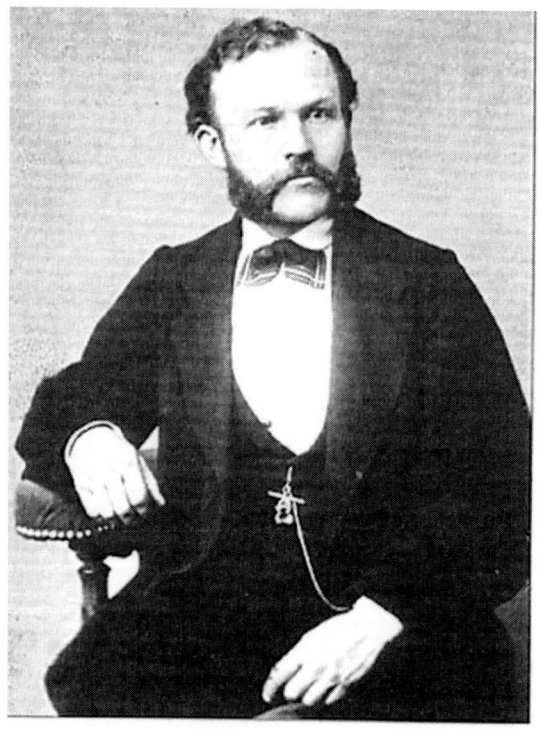

Figure 11.3
Ferdinand Adolf Kehrer (1837-1914).
In 1881 he used a transverse incision and performed what is, in essence, the modern lower uterine segment caesarean section

The modern era of lower uterine segment caesarean section began in 1881 and the architect was Ferdinand Adolf Kehrer (1837-1914), Professor of Obstetrics at Heidelberg, Germany. (Figure 11.3) He chose to perform the caesarean section with a transverse incision in the uterus just above the cervix – as Johnson had proposed some one hundred years earlier. His first patient had a contracted pelvis due to osteomalacia and had been in obstructed labour for thirty hours. Her abode was a small cottage in the village of Meckelsheim, near Heidelberg and the operation took place there on 25th September 1881. A translation of his operative description follows:[3,5]

'Preliminary preparations were then made. Two hanging lamps, one stand lamp, and several candlesticks were assembled, a small table made ready with a stool at the end of it to support the legs, the instruments laid out in carbolic water, and the hand spray fitted up. Chloroform was administered and the patient brought to the table. The genitalia were shaved, the abdominal wall and thighs washed with carbolic solution, the vagina douched and then packed with a swab wrung out of the same lotion. The abdominal wall was incised in the linea alba below the umbilicus. The uterine wall was divided a little above the floor of the uterovesical pouch, the infant's left ear then presenting in the wound. The latter was now enlarged laterally as far as the round ligaments on either side. The head was delivered by applying the fingers of both hands as one would use the forceps. The placenta was extracted by drawing on the cord.'

Kehrer placed great emphasis on the 'doppelnaht' (double layer) closure of the uterine incision, (Figure 11.4).

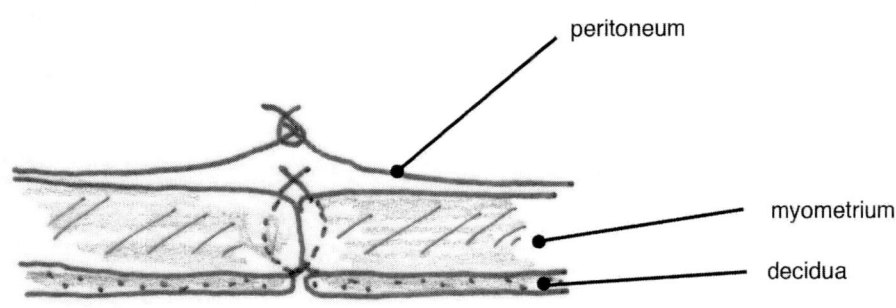

Figure 11.4
Kehrer's 'doppelnaht' (double layer) suture closure of the lower transverse uterine incision

By placing the incision transversely in the lower uterine segment the visceral (utero-vesical) peritoneal layer was easily separated from the underlying muscle. He used six silk sutures to close the full thickness of uterine muscle and twelve to unite the peritoneum. Both mother and infant survived. He later advocated the use of a continuous suture to close the peritoneum. Kehrer felt that separation of the peritoneum from the uterine muscle allowed this layer to avoid disruption by retraction and involution of the underlying muscle and thus maintain its integrity, thereby preventing infected lochia that might seep through the uterine muscle wall from entering the peritoneal cavity.[3] He also reasoned that the transverse incision in the lower uterine segment was less likely to gape and therefore easier to close than the classical upper uterine incision - as it proved to be. Kehrer performed a second caesarean with this technique on 13th November 1881 – the infant lived but the mother died.

Both Kehrer and Sanger stressed the technique of uterine closure in their publications [3,7] (see chapter 9). Kehrer's paper preceded that of Sanger by a few weeks and described the results of the two caesareans performed; whereas Sanger's publication was theoretical and he did not carry out his own procedure for another two years. However, Sanger forcefully and energetically promoted his technique of uterine closure and it was adopted with success by others who were used to the simpler classical upper segment incision. Thus it was Sanger's technique of classical caesarean section that held sway through the latter part of the 19th century and into the early 20th century.[8]

In many ways Kehrer has not received appropriate acknowledgement of his ground-breaking innovation; namely, improving the short and long term integrity of the uterine scar by a simple and logical approach that remains the basis of the transverse lower segment caesarean operation some 135 years later. Adolf Kehrer did not live to see widespread acceptance of his procedure, but his son, a Professor of Medicine at Marburg did, and in 1929 was able to say with pride:[5]

'The birthplace of abdominal caesarean section is a lowly cottage in the village of Meckesheim, near Heidelberg, and its birthday is the 25th of September, 1881'

By the end of the 19th century good results were being reported using the classical caesarean operation, provided it was performed electively or in early labour before intrauterine infection set in. However, septic cases with neglected or obstructed labour continued to have a high maternal death rate – such that fetal destructive operations or caesarean hysterectomy might be chosen over the more conservative classical caesarean section.[2] As a solution to this conundrum the main elements of Kehrer's operation were revived in 1906 by Fritz Frank (1856-1923). As a young obstetrician Frank had spent time as a junior assistant in Kehrer's department, before his appointment as Director of the School of Midwifery in Cologne, Germany.

Frank used a transverse suprapubic incision to cut through all layers of the abdominal wall, including the parietal peritoneum (Baudenhauer's incision). Like Kehrer, he separated the utero-vesical (visceral) peritoneum from the lower uterine segment and divided this transversely. He then sutured together, with continuous catgut, the upper edges of the parietal and visceral peritoneum – attempting to block the exposed lower uterine segment from the general peritoneal cavity. Then, as Kehrer had done, he opened the lower uterine segment transversely and delivered the infant *'.....with the help of extra-abdominal pressure.....'* [2,5,9] In the early cases Frank placed an iodoform gauze drain from the uterine wound through the cervix to the vagina; he later stopped this component of the operation. He used continuous catgut sutures for both the peritoneum and uterine muscle closure. The thin muscle of the lower uterine segment, passive during the puerperium, was amenable to easy closure with catgut, in contrast to the thick and actively contracting and retracting upper uterine segment.

Frank conceived his operation as an alternative to the Porro caesarean hysterectomy for infected cases:[5,9]

'I hold my method to be an essential advance, for by proceeding in this way, the woman is spared much loss of blood, peritonitis is prevented, and the operator is permitted greater latitude with regard to the time when intervention is decided upon.'

By 1907 Frank reported thirteen successful cases – all in women infected after prolonged labour; the very cases in which, at that time, caesarean hysterectomy was advised because of the high maternal death rate with septic cases delivered by classical caesarean section. To achieve these results and preserve the uterus in these infected women was a huge advance and helped establish the role of the lower uterine segment caesarean section in Continental Europe. As Frank proudly wrote:[5,9]

'Wir opfern nicht, sondern wir retten sie beide'
(We don't sacrifice them, but we save them both)

The years following Frank's impressive results saw increased acceptance of the lower segment caesarean over the then well established classical caesarean section. Virtually the entire development of the lower segment operation through the 19th century had been carried out in Germany.

By the early 20th century series from France, Italy, Britain and the USA reported the successful adoption of the lower segment caesarean – particularly in infected or potentially infected cases.[2,5] Much of this work was within the historical background of the First World War, when the exchange of academic information was suspended.

Eardley Lancelot Holland (1879-1967), obstetrician at the London Hospital, was the first to undertake a comprehensive study of the results of caesarean section across the hospitals of Britain and Ireland. Holland was a medical officer in France in the First World War and had studied in Berlin in 1929. He was later to become president of the Royal College of Obstetricians and Gynaecologists and be knighted for his services. In an extensive review of the early experience with the lower segment operation in Britain and Ireland from 1911 to 1920 involving some four thousand cases Holland summarised the advantages as follows:[10]

1. *'The wound lies in a quiet part of the uterus, and is at rest during healing. There is no tendency for the edges of the wound to be drawn apart, or for gaps to be formed between the sutures. For these reasons healing occurs in more favourable circumstances than in the classical operation.*
2. *The uterine incision is made through a less vascular area, and bleeding from the edges is extremely slight.*
3. *The edges of the wound are thin; suture is therefore easier and quicker.*
4. *The position of the wound is such that adhesions to the intestines, omentum, or abdominal wall cannot occur; there is only a short line of peritoneal sutures at the bottom of the utero-vesical pouch.*
5. *The uterine wound is covered with a thick layer of fascia and by the bladder, and perfect closure of the peritoneum can be made. For those reasons there is less likelihood of infection of the peritoneal cavity; for it is generally conceded that the source of peritoneal infection is not so much due to contamination by liquor amnii or other uterine contents during the operation as to the subsequent passage of infection from the uterine cavity between the edges of the incision. Should peritoneal infection occur the lower abdomen is more resistant than the upper.*
6. *The operation causes less disturbance of the abdominal contents; the intestines are never seen.*
7. *The scar is in a safer area for subsequent pregnancy and labour, for the lower uterine segment stretches late in labour. The stretching to which the scar is subjected is purely passive, for there is no powerful active drag upon each side of the scar, as there is in the scar of the classical operation.*
8. *As regards the performance of the operation, it is just as easy to a practiced surgeon as the Classical; true, there is more "operating" in it – it is not done, as it were, by two strokes of the knife, as is the Classical. The more advanced the patient is in labour, the easier will*

the operation be and the lower will the incision lie in the lower segment and cervix; in fact, in cases of excessive retraction of the uterus, the incision will lie partly in the upper end of the vagina.

9. *So far only one case of ruptured scar has been reported, and this is not a fair case, as the upper end of the incision had to be extended upwards on to the body of the uterus. At the same time it must be remembered that very few lower segment operations have been done compared to the many thousands by the classical method.'*

Holland found that the risk of uterine rupture in a pregnancy or labour following classical caesarean section was 4%.[11] Subsequent experience showed this to be about ten times the risk of lower segment caesarean rupture.

In contrast to Kehrer and Frank, a number of obstetricians used a vertical incision in the lower segment – the rationale being a perceived reduced risk of bleeding from lateral extension of the transverse incision. Bernard Krönig (1863-1918), from Freiburg, Germany, favoured the vertical incision, *'der cervicale Kaiserschnitt,'* but felt the most important aspect was low entry through the utero-vesical peritoneum and downward retraction of the bladder, so that the uterine incision was placed to lie behind the bladder.[12] Others, including Kerr, Marshall and St George Wilson in Britain, and Doerfler in Germany, used the transverse uterine incision.[5,13,14]

Support for the transverse incision was provided by the histological work of H. Goerttler of Kiel in 1930; he showed that the muscle fibres in the cervix, and in the lower uterine segment were arranged in a circular manner.[5] The New York obstetrician, Alfred Beck (1886-1979), introduced the lower segment operation, based on Kronig's technique, to the United States in 1919.[15] Joseph B DeLee (1869-1942), the influential Professor of Obstetrics at Northwestern University, Chicago, was an early and strong proponent of the lower segment operation and favoured the vertical uterine incision which he called *'laparotrachelotomy.'* [8,16,17] The argument of those who used the transverse incision was that the vertical incision sometimes extended into the upper uterine segment and would therefore be more prone to subsequent rupture; and that extension of the vertical incision downwards could injure the bladder.[5]

By the mid 20th century the transverse lower segment incision became the accepted choice. In addition to the other benefits of the lower segment incision, all obstetricians emphasised, as had Kehrer, that watertight closure of the utero-vesical peritoneum was the key to preventing any seepage of infected material through the uterine incision from entering the peritoneal cavity. Alfred Beck closed the utero-vesical peritoneal layer by suturing one flap over the other to ensure the integrity of this seal.[18] The uterine muscle was closed in two layers of continuous sutures. If the muscle layer was very thin, as it often was in advanced labour, it was closed in one layer and a second layer of muscle folded over the first with a Lembert type of suture.

By the late 1930s Marshall was able to report the results of 1,263 lower segment caesareans in nine hospitals in Britain, with a maternal mortality of 1.4%.[5] Edwin Daily and Joseph DeLee, both from Chicago, reported similar results from five hundred and 1,875 cases respectively with maternal mortality rates of 1%.[5,19] Thus the results of the lower segment operation with infected patients were comparable to those of classical caesarean section in uninfected women. This compared to maternal death rates of 5-8% for classical caesarean section in infected cases.

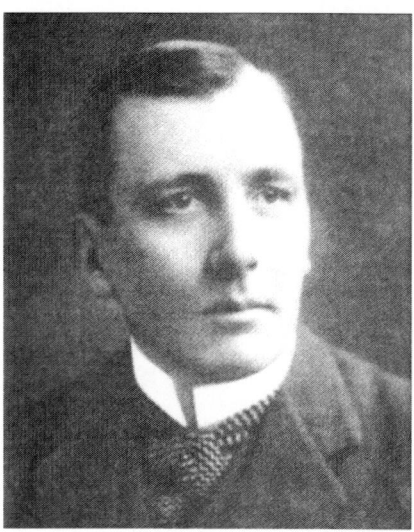

Figure 11.5
Munro Kerr (1868-1960)
Helped establish the transverse lower segment incision as the standard technique of caesarean section

In Britain, Munro Kerr of Glasgow did more than any other obstetrician to advance the case for the lower segment operation, along with Marshall and Wilson of Liverpool.[5,14] Kerr, who had been involved with Holland in the review of cases of uterine rupture after classical caesarean section,[10,11] did his first lower segment caesarean in 1911 and reported his results in the 1920s and 30s.[13,20] (Figure 11.5) His main argument in favour of the lower segment caesarean was the stronger uterine scar with less likelihood of rupture in a subsequent pregnancy. As he wrote:[13]

'I make no claims to originality as regards the incision, and I recommend it

only because I believe that the cicatrix that results will be less liable to rupture. The advantages of the incision are that one cuts through a less vascular area; the bleeding is extraordinarily slight unless the wound is allowed to extend into the vessels at the side. In the second place, it is thin and consequently the surfaces can be readily brought together......The third advantage, and it is a very important one, is that the wound in this area is at rest during the early days of the puerperium. Lastly, there is this great advantage that owing to the fact that the lower uterine segment does not become fully stretched until labour is well advanced the scar is in a safer region than the ordinary longitudinal one.'

For many years he was a lone voice in Britain promoting the lower segment procedure over the classical caesarean section. Acceptance came slowly in the conservative world of British obstetrics - but it did come. In 1949, at the 12th British Congress of Obstetrics and Gynaecology, held in London several years after Kerr had retired from clinical practice, he was summoned to the lecture stage to receive plaudits for his role in popularising the lower segment operation. With his usual flair for the dramatic he faced the audience, raised his arms and declared: *'Alleluia! The strife is o'er, the battle done!'* [8,21]

REFERENCES

1. Johnson RW. A New System of Midwifery. 2nd edition. London: D. Wilson and G. Nichol;1786.
2. Young JH. Caesarean Section: the History and Development of the Operation from Earliest Times. London: HK Lewis & Co Ltd; 1944. p190-221.
3. Kehrer FA. Über ein modificirtes Verfahren beim Kaiserschnitte. Arch Gynakol 1882;19:177-209.
4. Osiander FB. Handbuch der Entbindungshurst. Vol 2.Tübingen: 1821.
5. Marshall CM. Caesarean Section: Lower Segment Operation. Bristol: John Wright & Sons Ltd;1939. p1-31.
6. Ricci JV. The Development of Gynaecological Surgery and Instruments. Philadelphia: The Blakistan Company; 1949. p184.
7. Sanger M. Der Kaiserschnitt. Arch Gynakol 1882;19:370-8.
8. Baskett TF. On the Shoulders of Giants: Eponyms and Names in Obstetrics and Gynaecology. Cambridge: Cambridge University Press; 2008.
9. Frank F. Suprasymphysere Entbindung und ihre Verhaltniss zu den anderen Operationen bei Engenen Becken.Arch Gynakol 1907;81:46-58.
10. Holland E. Methods of performing caesarean section. J Obstet Gynaecol Br Emp. 1921;28:349-446.
11. Holland E. Rupture of the caesarean scar in subsequent pregnancy or labour. J Obstet Gynaecol Br Emp 1921:28:488-522.

12. Kronig B. Transperitonealer Cervikaler Kaiserschnitt. In: Doderlein A, Kronig B. Operative Gynakologie. 1912. p879-87.
13. Kerr JM. The lower uterine segment incision in conservative caesarean section. J Obstet Gynaecol Br Emp 1921;28:475-87.
14. Wilson JStG. Lower uterine segment caesarean section. J Obstet Gynaecol Br Emp 1931;38:504-15.
15. Beck AC. Observations on a series of cases of caesarean section done at the Long Island Hospital during the past six years. Am J Obstet Dis Women Child 1919;79:197-14.
16. DeLee JB, Cornell EL. Low cervical cesarean section. (laparo-trachelotomy) JAMA 1922;79:109-14.
17. DeLee JB. An illustrated history of the low or cervical cesarean section. Am J Obstet Gynecol 1925;10:503-20.
18. Beck AC. The advantages and disadvantages of the two-flap low incision cesarean section, with a report of eighty-three cases done by fifteen operators. Am J Obstet Gynecol 1921;1:586-94.
19. Daily EF. Cesarean section: An analysis of five hundred consecutive operations. Am J Obstet Gynecol 1935;30:204-8.
20. Kerr JM. Caesarean section. Proc R Soc Med 1936;29:1645-51.
21. Baskett TF, Calder AA, Arulkumaran S (eds). Munro Kerr's Operative Obstetrics. 12th edition. Edinburgh: Elsevier; 2014. p132-144.

Chapter 12

Caesarean hysterectomy

On 21st July, 1869 the first caesarean hysterectomy was performed as an act of unplanned desperation.[1] The obstetric surgeon was Horatio Storer (1830-1922) of Boston who had graduated in both medicine and law at Harvard University and was professor of obstetrics and medical jurisprudence at the Berkshire Medical School.[2] (Figure 12.1)

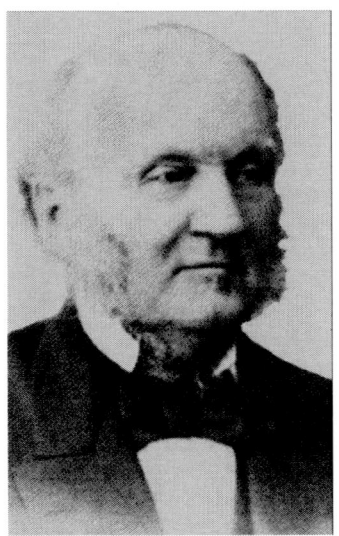

Figure 12.1
Horatio Storer (1830-1922)
In 1869 Storer performed the first caesarean hysterectomy - not by choice!

The patient, Mrs H, was a thirty-seven year old primigravida in labour with a fixed pelvic mass obstructing vaginal delivery and precluding '..... *any other mechanical interference per vaginam.*' Storer's plan was to perform the minimum surgery necessary to relieve the obstruction and then allow labour and vaginal delivery. However, at laparotomy under chloroform anaesthesia he found, not the removable ovarian tumour he had hoped for, but a fibroid tumour of the lower uterine segment. Attempted excision of the fibroid was attended by considerable bleeding so *'Dr Storer extended his incision into the cavity of the uterus and with all expedition removed a male child, weighing eight pounds; it being, as well as the placenta, in an advanced state of decomposition.....'.* At this point the haemorrhage was described as *'perfectly frightful'* so Storer was forced, *'with his usual self-possession'*, to proceed to a subtotal hysterectomy. The cervical stump was doubly ligated and *'seared by the hot iron.'* The operation lasted three hours.[1] The case was subsequently presented to the Boston Gynaecological Society and published in their proceedings, not by Storer, but by his assistant George Bixby.[1]

Before Storer's harrowing surgical encounter a number of physicians experimented with caesarean hysterectomy in animals, given the almost universally fatal outcome of caesarean section with retention of the uterus. The first was Giuseppe Cavallini of Florence who, in 1768, after experiments that involved removing the gravid uterus of dogs and sheep, concluded [3]:

'I do not doubt that the uterus is not at all necessary to life; but whether it may be plucked out with impunity from the human body we cannot be certain without a further series of experiments of this kind which perhaps a more fortunate generation will obtain.'

James Blundell (1790-1878), a lecturer in midwifery and physiology at St Thomas' and Guy's hospitals, London, was one of the next generation to carry these experiments further.[2] His own surgical experiments on pregnant rabbits convinced him that laparotomy and removal of the gravid uterus need not be fatal. He concluded that the amount of wounded and infected tissue (ie the uterus) left behind after caesarean section was a greater source of fatal haemorrhage and infection than if the uterus was entirely removed.[4] As he said in one of his lectures on obstetrics at Guy's Hospital in 1828 [5]:

'In speculative moments, I have sometimes felt inclined to persuade myself that the dangers of the caesarean operation might be considerably diminished by removal of the uterus. Perhaps this method of operating may prove an eminent and valuable improvement.'

It was to be almost fifty years before Blundell's speculation was put to the test in the clinical arena. Edoardo Porro (1842-1902) was a thoughtful obstetrician and the Professor of Obstetrics at the University of Pavia. (Figure 12.2) At that time no woman in Pavia had survived caesarean delivery and Porro himself had operated in 1871 with a fatal result to the mother, although the infant survived [2]. After review of this and other cases Porro, like Blundell before him, concluded that the mortal outcome of caesarean section was due to haemorrhage and sepsis originating from the retained uterus.[2] He also carried out experiments excising the uterus of pregnant rabbits, as well as removing the uterus of human cadavers in preparation for his first caesarean hysterectomy.

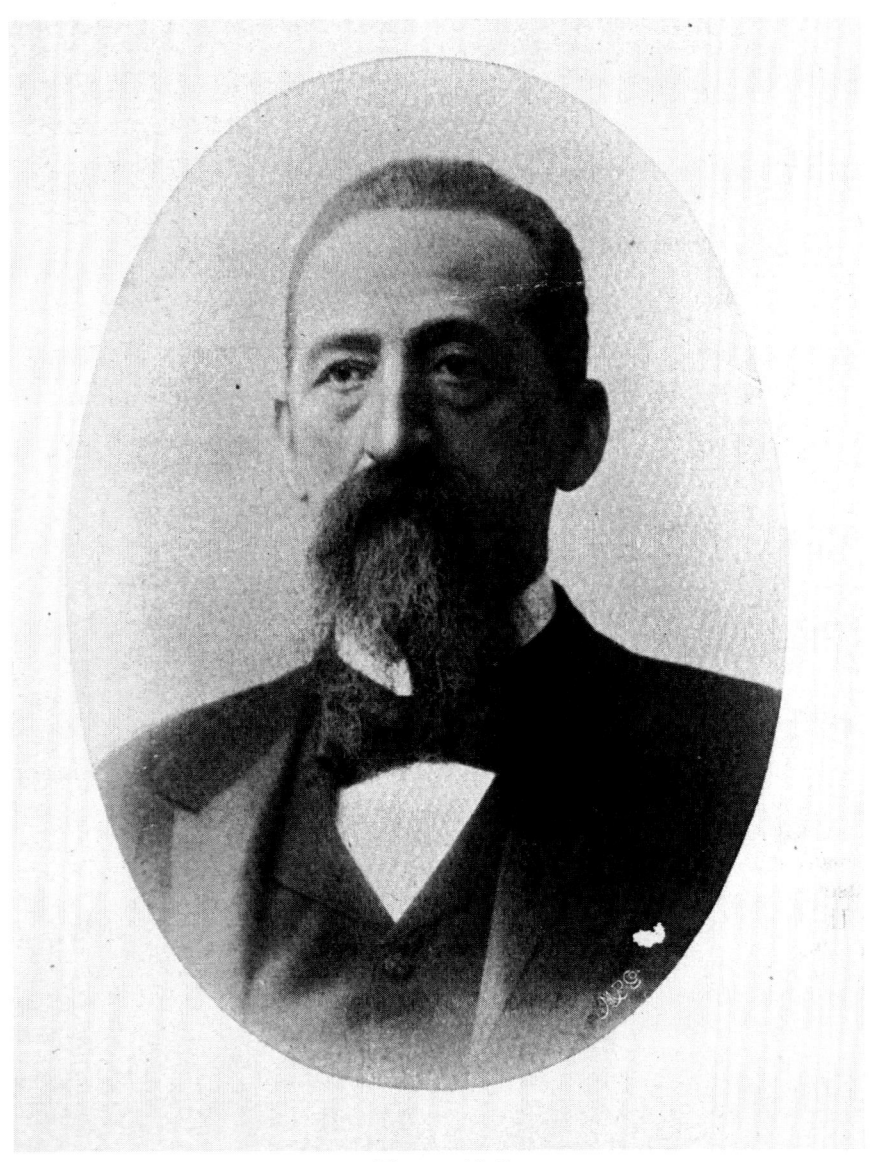

Figure 12.2
Edoardo Porro (1842-1902)
In 1876, after careful planning and preparation, Porro carried out the first of a series of successful caesarean hysterectomies.

The opportunity came on 21st May 1876 when he encountered a twenty-five year old rachitic primigravida – ironically by the name of Julia Cavallini. She had a distorted pelvis with a true obstetric conjugate of four centimetres. After seven hours of labour she was given chloroform anaesthesia and Porro delivered the baby by caesarean section. Then, using a metal snare *('serre noeud')* he encircled the lower uterus and excised the uterus, tubes and ovaries. The cervical stump was fixed through the lower end of the abdominal incision, thus exteriorising any potential septic discharge from the cervix. A drain was then placed through the Pouch of Douglas into the vagina. Post operatively she received champagne and laudanum, was pronounced *'cured'* in forty days and left the hospital with her infant as the first woman to survive caesarean section in Pavia. [3,6,7]

Peter Müller (1836-1922), Professor of Obstetrics at Berne, Switzerland suggested a minor modification to Porro's operation. He brought the uterus out of the abdominal cavity and put an elastic tourniquet around its base before making the uterine incision. This, he argued, would reduce bleeding and avoid the spill of the uterine contents into the peritoneal cavity.[8] The drawbacks were the large abdominal incision and the potential, and in some cases real danger of fetal asphyxiation from the elastic tourniquet. The maternal results were about the same as the Porro technique and, because of the fetal risks it was mainly used in cases where the fetus was already dead.[3]

The Porro operation, as it came to be known, was slowly embraced by a number of surgeons in Europe and to a limited degree in Britain and the United States.[9] While it may seem radical, and it was, it has to be put in the context of the high maternal mortality associated with caesarean delivery in the early/mid 19th century. [10] For example, in the maternity hospitals of both Paris and Vienna in the one hundred years preceding Porro's operation, no mother had survived caesarean section. [3,7] By 1884, Clement Godson of the City of London Lying-in Hospital tabulated 134 cases of the Porro operation that had been performed in Europe and the USA. The maternal mortality was 56%; but this had fallen from 85.7% in 1877 to 35.7% in 1883; a considerable improvement on the death rate for caesarean section without hysterectomy.[3,11] Porro himself had operated five times with four mothers saved. [11] Between 1885 and 1889 there were 158 cases in all countries and the maternal mortality had dropped to 29%.[3]

Godson's comprehensive review of the world experience with the Porro operation also included details of his own case in 1882 – the first in Britain with maternal survival.[11] As an account of major obstetric surgery one hundred and thirty-five years ago, some of the details warrant review. The woman was small, 4ft 4in with a pelvic deformity associated with childhood trauma, such that her true obstetric conjugate was only three centimetres. Intercourse had occurred once only, so the gestation was known and the operation was scheduled for thirty-eight weeks – 27th November 1882. Half-an-ounce of beef extract was given six hours before the operation, followed by a soap and water enema. Inhalation anaesthesia was given with nitrous oxide and ether. The bladder was emptied with a catheter. The midline sub-umbilical abdominal incision was made under the Lister principle with carbolic acid spray. *'The uterine incision was made, at about the junction of the lower with the middle third – just large enough to admit the finger.....I immediately inserted the tips of each fore-finger, and tore the womb open transversely'.*[11] Godson listed the times for each component of the operation:

- Start of abdominal incision to delivery of the infant: 8 minutes
- Application of uterine encircling snare (serre noeud): 2 minutes
- Excision of uterus, tubes and ovaries: 10 minutes
- Stitching of abdominal wound, including cervical stump: 22 minutes

The infant was a girl *'unusually large (8½ lb), vigorous and well nourished'.*

Post-operative care included regular administration of rectal opium and, interestingly, she was *'placed on a water bed to avoid bed sores.'*[11]

She was discharged 30 days later. By chance, Godson met her eight months later when he noted *'She was in perfect health and said she had never felt better in her life.'*

Another contentious surgical point of caesarean hysterectomy was whether to leave the cervical stump in the pelvis or exteriorise it by suturing it into the lower part of the abdominal incision. Godson reviewed this factor in his report of 134 cases; the lower maternal death rate in those with exteriorisation of the cervical stump (53%) compared to those with the stump dropped into the pelvis (73%), confirmed the majority opinion at that time.[11]

One factor, not mentioned in any of the reports in the 19th century on the Porro operation, was the longer term effects of removal of the ovaries in young women. They would have experienced an abrupt surgical menopause and must have suffered considerably from the acute and chronic effects of oestrogen deprivation. Presumably, survival was enough for the operation to be declared a success and/or there was no follow up – beyond survival.

One of the pleasures of delving into old papers on a subject is the discovery of whimsical case reports. One such epic surgical and naval encounter was reported by Donald Roy, a surgeon with obstetric training, who served during the First World War on the Royal Naval hospital ship *'Plassy'* at Scapa Flow in the remote waters of the Orkney Islands off the coast of Scotland.[12] Here, on 14th October, 1915, *'Owing to the death of the local doctor, the medical care of the civilian population had been taken over by the navy......'* Roy *' was called in consultation to see an achondroplastic dwarf primigravida, aged 21, who had been forty-eight hours in labour which had become obstructed '* The case report continued:[12]

' The house was about two miles from the ship by water and fortunately the

weather was good.....The patient was lying in one of the cupboard beds usual in the islands, which are more adapted to shutting out the searching winds of the island than to obstetrical manipulations. On examination, she was found to be a dwarf of very small size (4ft 2½ in). Her condition was fairly satisfactory considering that she had been in labour forty-eight hours. Her temperature was 100.4 °F., her pulse 108. She was considerably demoralized, and, in common with the rest of the family, had made up her mind that her only delivery would be by the hand of death......Vaginal examination showed a leg and the cord down in the vagina; the cord was not pulsating, the leg was beginning to desquamate. The child had evidently been dead some time. It was obviously a very small pelvis, as the promontory of the sacrum was met with almost as soon as the finger entered the vagina.....the true conjugate was calculated to be 1¾ inches, and there was also less well-marked contraction of the transverse diameter at the brim. It was fairly evident at once that any variety of embryotomy was out of the question...... It was therefore decided to remove the patient to the hospital ship "Plassy" for Caesarean section. After a good deal of pressure the relatives abandoned their fatalistic attitude and consented to this being done. This removal would have been possible only during the fine weather which fortunately prevailed at the time. It had to be done in three stages, and of course no lights could be shown. First, the patient had to be carried in the dark along two or three hundred yards of rocky beach to a rough landing-place where a small dingy could be brought in. She then had to be rowed out to the motor boat and transferred thereto, carried two miles by water to the ship, and hauled on board in the special tray used for this purpose, which is lowered from the ship's winch, and the cot and patient placed on it and slung on board. .....An anaesthetic was given.....Caesarean section was decided upon. There was evidently an added risk of sepsis owing to the length of time the woman had been in labour and the examinations made. Further, the relatives and the patient herself were anxious that she should be sterilized in view of the great risk of another labour should she again become pregnant in that isolated spot, practically cut off for weeks at a time in bad weather from the main island. A long septic puerperium could not be risked as the ship might be ordered away at any time in the next fourteen days. Taking these three considerations into account. I decided if possible to remove the uterus and its contents unopened, leaving the tubes and ovaries behind.'

Roy eventually did a caesarean section followed by subtotal hysterectomy with preservation of the tubes and ovaries. After which: *'The patient made a rapid recovery and sailed away in her father's boat to her home on the fourteenth day, just before the ship left the Flow..... the patient reported herself quite well at Christmas 1915.'*

This was: '…..*the only recorded case of Caesarean section performed in the Navy Medical Service. It caused considerable interest in the Fleet, and gave rise to some ribald jests from senior officers of the combatant branch.*' [12]

Thus concluded the low-key account of what must have been a dramatic, prolonged and exhausting episode – not least for the patient.

In its time Porro's caesarean hysterectomy, by removing the septic focus in the infected patient, reduced maternal mortality compared to caesarean section alone. It was, however, a radical and mutilating operation removing any chance of future pregnancy and with the attendant side effects of castration. By the late 19th century it was supplanted by the classical caesarean technique of Sanger (see chapter 9), with which maternal death rates between 6 and 12% were achieved in Germany and Britain.[3] Porro's operation continued to be used, but only in cases with marked intrauterine sepsis at the time of caesarean section, such as the one detailed above.

With the development of anaesthesia, blood transfusion and antibiotics the safety of both caesarean section and caesarean hysterectomy improved dramatically by the mid 20th century; to the extent that elective caesarean hysterectomy was considered by some to be appropriate for sterilisation purposes. In 1951, the influential Edward Davis of the Chicago Lying-in Hospital wrote of caesarean hysterectomy as '*A logical advance in modern obstetric surgery*'.[13] He felt that it was indicated if sterilisation was desired, if there was disease (usually fibroids) or '*excess scarring*' of the uterus and '*in women near the end of their reproductive period, in whom the uterus no longer serves a useful function*'.[13] Davis also advocated total over subtotal hysterectomy because of potential problems with the retained cervix: development of cancer, dyspareunia and prolapse. Although in the pre-cervical cancer screening era it was estimated that 500 to 1000 hysterectomies would be required to prevent one case of cervical cancer.[14] A review of 1000 cases of caesarean hysterectomy from 1938 to 1957 at the New Orleans Charity Hospital represented 15% of all caesarean sections at that hospital. Despite the high morbidity (49%) the author felt the operation was no more risky than caesarean section alone.[15] Others contested this conclusion and found that the maternal morbidity with caesarean hysterectomy was higher than with caesarean section and tubal ligation.[14,16] By the late 1960s mainstream obstetric opinion was that elective caesarean hysterectomy solely for sterilisation was not advised.[7]

Caesarean hysterectomy continues to be needed in modern obstetrics for rare obstetric emergencies. There is an association between caesarean section and the need for hysterectomy in both the index and the previous pregnancy, and with rising caesarean section rates the incidence of caesarean hysterectomy is increasing.[17,18] The main indications are abnormal placentation (placenta praevia and/or accreta), uterine rupture and uterine atony refractory to oxytocic drugs in the exhausted and infected uterus associated with prolonged obstructed labour.[17] A recent ten year review (2001-2010) found a maternal mortality range from 0-24%, with the worst rates occurring in areas with limited health services – not a lot different from the figures of the late 19th century.[19]

REFERENCES

1. Bixby GH. Extirpation of the puerperal uterus by abdominal section. J Gynaecol Soc Boston 1869;1:223-32.
2. Baskett TF. On the Shoulders of Giants: Eponyms and Names in Obstetrics and Gynaecology. 2nd edition. Cambridge: Cambridge University Press; 2008.
3. Young JH. Caesarean Section: The History and Development of the Operation from Earliest Times. London: HK Lewis and Co Ltd; 1944, p93-107, 142-4.
4. Blundell J. Researches Physiological and Pathological: Instituted Principally With a View to the Improvement of Medical and Surgical Practice. London: E. Cox and Son; 1824 p23-27,61-2.
5. Blundell J. Lectures at Guy's Hospital. Lancet 1828;2:163-67.
6. Porro E. Della amputazione utero-ovarica come complemento di taglio cesareo. Ann Univ Med Chir (Milan) 1876;237:289-350.
7. Durfee RB. Evolution of cesarean hysterectomy. Clin Obstet Gynecol 1969;12:575-89.
8. Müller P. Ein Kaiserschnitt mit extirpation des uterus. Zentralbl Gynakol 1878;2:97-104.
9. Todman D. Eduardo Porro (1842-1902) and the development of caesarean section: a reappraisal. Internet J Gynecol Obstet 2006, Vol 7, No2.
10. Sparic R, Kadija S, Hudelist G, Glisic A, Buzadzic S. History of caesarean hysterectomy. ACI/IZ Istorije Hirurgije 2012;59:9-12.
11. Godson C. Porro's operation. BMJ 1884;1:142-59.
12. Roy DW. Caesarean hysterectomy for obstructed labour on board a Royal Naval hospital ship during the Great War. J Obstet Gynaecol Br Emp 1921;28:554-8.
13. Davis ME. Complete cesarean hysterectomy: A logical advance in modern obstetric surgery. Am J Obstet Gynecol 1951;62:838-53.
14. O'Leary JA, Steer CM. A 10 year review of cesarean hysterectomy. Am J Obstet Gynecol 1964;90:227-31.
15. Barclay DL. Cesarean hysterectomy at the Charity Hospital in New Orleans – 1000 consecutive operations. Clin Obstet Gynecol 1969;12:635-51
16. Pletsch TD, Sandberg EG. Cesarean hysterectomy for sterilization. Am J Obstet Gynecol 1963;85:254-9.
17. Baskett TF. Emergency obstetric hysterectomy. J Obstet Gynaecol

2003;23:353-5.
18. Wen SW, Huang L, Liston RM, Heaman M, Baskett TF, Rusen ID. Severe maternal morbidity in Canada 1991-2001. Can Med Assoc J 2005;173:759-61.
19. Baskett TF. Peripartum hysterectomy. In: Arulkumaran S, Karoski M, Keith LG, Lalonde AB., B-Lynch C, (eds). A Comprehensive Textbook of Postpartum Haermorrhage. 2nd Edition. Duncow: Sapiens Publishing. 2012.pp 462-5.

Chapter 13

Anaesthesia for caesarean delivery

Before effective methods of pain relief were developed women undergoing caesarean section had, of necessity, to follow the *'grin and bear it'* or *'pull yourself together'* schools of suffering. Or as Louis Velpeau (1795-1867) of the Charité Hospital in Paris put it, *'…..a great degree of resignation, such as is pretty often observed in country-people, is most of all to be desired.'* [1] Thus, early descriptions of caesarean delivery advised tying the patient to the bed or table in order to prevent her moving during the operation. Others suggested the use of assistants to restrain the woman, feeling this was more humane than binding her down: *'…..she must be secured by several assistants, who are to hold her hands, thighs and even the body, to spare her the horrors of being tied down.'* [2]

James Blundell, the London obstetrician, had a more optimistic view of the resolve of women facing caesarean section:[3]

'Women possessing perhaps a larger share of passive courage than men, we may, I believe, generally trust to their fortitude; and I deem it, therefore, unnecessary to alarm by the use of ligatures, though a steady assistant, of firm nerves, ought to stand on either side, in readiness to secure the patient, should her resolution fail.'

Bloodletting

For centuries, up to the 19th century, bloodletting was prescribed for just about any medical misdemeanor, so it is no surprise that it would be tried to relieve the pain of surgical procedures. The principle was to drain enough blood from the circulation to produce syncope – know as 'ad deliquium animi' (to failure of life).[4] This proved successful for short procedures such as the reduction of joint dislocations. It was used by some physicians, notably Benjamin Rush and William Dewees of Philadelphia, to induce syncope and thus relieve, albeit temporarily, the pain of labour.[4] The same approach was taken to provide analgesia and muscle relaxation, via syncope, to facilitate procedures such as internal version and breech extraction. However, there is no reference to its use for caesarean section.

Analgesic drugs

Since the Hippocratic era attempts were made to relieve pain with plant derivatives such as mandrake, alcohol, cannabis, hyoscyamus (henbane) and opium – sometimes known as the anodynes of antiquity.[5] In the middle ages a number of these agents were combined: opium, mandrake, henbane, hemlock, blackberries and lettuce seeds, which mixture was soaked in a sea sponge and allowed to dry – *spongia somnifera*. When needed, the sponge was dipped in water, held to the patients nostrils and inhaled before surgery.[4] Early botanical and pharmaceutical texts tended to extol the qualities of the anodynes of antiquity as potential analgesic aids to surgery, but the surgical texts rarely mentioned them.[6] Indeed, modern experiments on animals show that soporific sponges were inadequate for surgical anaesthesia,[7] and there is no record of them being used for caesarean section.

Of all the ancient anodynes only opium derivatives continue to be used for pain relief. Until injection became available, in 1853, the most common oral opium administration was laudanum – the alcoholic tincture of opium to which saffron, cinnamon and cloves were added for taste.[8] It soon became apparent that this was not adequate for surgical anaesthesia, although it was of benefit for postoperative pain relief. This was summarised by the Glasgow born, London-based surgeon James Moore (1763-1834) in 1784.[4,8]

'Opium.....is highly expedient to abate the smarting of the wound after the operation is over, and to induce sleep; but the strongest dose we dare venture to give has little or no effect in mitigating the suffering of the patient during the operation.'

In 1805 Friedrich Serterner (1783-1841), a pharmacist's apprentice in Germany, isolated the active principle of opium, which he named 'morphium' after the Greek god of dreams.[8] After the development of the hypodermic needle and syringe in 1853, by Alexander Wood of Edinburgh (1817-1884), morphine became the most commonly used opium alkaloid.[8]

However, there is scant mention of either laudanum or morphine being used to alleviate the pain of caesarean section – perhaps because in the pre-anaesthetic era the operation was usually performed when the woman was almost moribund and beyond analgesic assistance.

Cold analgesia

The effect of cold in reducing the sensation in tissues was applied by Napoleon's Surgeon-in-Chief, Dominique Jean Larrey (1766-1842), during the retreat of the French army from Russia in 1812.[9] He noted the reduction of pain during amputation in freezing temperatures and advocated this technique to reduce surgical pain. This principle was later applied using ether or ethyl chloride sprays to freeze and numb the tissues.[10,11] Mostly used for dental analgesia, it was also tried for abdominal incisions and, as Playfair wrote in 1876, it had at least occasional use as an alternative to general anaesthesia for caesarean section: '......*local anaesthesia has been used by means of two spray producers acting simultaneously......if the patient has sufficient fortitude to dispense with general anaesthesia.*'[12] The wording suggests its efficacy in relieving the pain of caesarean section was limited – as one might expect. Thomas Radford of Manchester described four cases in which ether-spray was used at caesarean section.[13] He found that '...... *the abdominal parietes were completely anaesthetised*' but that the effect on the uterus was less predictable and could induce a sustained uterine contraction making extraction of the fetus difficult.[13]

Inhalation/General anaesthesia

Ether

William Morton (1819-1868) first demonstrated the use of ether on the 16th of October 1846 at the Massachusetts General Hospital in Boston. The surgeon was John Warren (1778-1856) who removed a vascular sub-mandibular tumour. Impressed with the anaesthetic Warren declared: '*Gentlemen, this is no humbug.*' Some three months later in Edinburgh on 19th January 1847, James Young Simpson (1811-1870), Professor of Midwifery, administered ether to a woman for labour and delivery – the first use of anaesthesia in childbirth.[14] While ether was effective it required a long time to induce anaesthesia and this, along with the pungent smell and respiratory irritation was distressing to patients. Simpson sought a better alternative and found it with chloroform.

Chloroform

Identified in 1831 independently by chemists in France, Germany and the USA, chloroform had the advantage of needing only small amounts to rapidly induce anaesthesia. In his quest for a superior inhalation anaesthetic Simpson had tested the effect of various promising agents on himself and colleagues at his house after dinner. In so doing the rapid effect of chloroform became apparent when he and two of his friends slipped unconscious beneath the dining room table shortly after inhaling the vapours from a glass of chloroform.[15] Four days later, on 8th November 1847, Simpson used chloroform to successfully ease the pain of labour and delivery in a doctor's wife to such good effect that she named the unfortunate child *'Anaesthesia.'* [16]

Nitrous oxide

Joseph Priestley (1733-1804), non-conformist clergyman and amateur scientist, identified nitrous oxide in 1772 and suggested that the medical profession explore its potential as a treatment for respiratory diseases, such as tuberculosis.[17] Humphrey Davy (1778-1829), working at the Medical Pneumatic Institution in Bristol, discovered the analgesic properties of nitrous oxide and suggested its use for surgical procedures as early as 1800.[18] This was ignored and the other qualities of intoxication and unprovoked, prolonged laughter resulted in nitrous oxide being used as a *'laughing gas'* at demonstrations and parties; until the mid 19th century when it was *'discovered'* as a dental anaesthetic. It became apparent that nitrous oxide administration produced hypoxia along with anaesthesia; thus it came to be given with oxygen. Stanislav Klikovich (1853-1910), a Polish physician, was the first to use inhalation of 80% nitrous oxide and 20% oxygen to relieve the pain of labour in 1881.[19,20]

Ether was the first general anaesthetic for caesarean section but was soon replaced by chloroform in many hospitals. Ether required such prolonged administration to achieve surgical anaesthesia that the fetus was often profoundly depressed at delivery. Herbert Spencer (1860-1941), the London obstetrician, in his personal series of 120 cases noted this effect: *'…..many of the children were asphyxiated and required a good deal of attention – not always harmless – to revive them.'* [21] As a result he changed his anaesthetic technique to start with rapid onset chloroform and continued with ether after the baby was delivered; which he felt should be done with considerable dispatch, *'The operation is then performed rapidly and the child is delivered in half a minute to a minute (once in eighteen seconds) from the commencement of the incision.'* [21] With this routine, neonatal asphyxia was avoided.

Different hospitals and anaesthetists developed their own techniques; often using nitrous oxide and/or chloroform to induce anaesthesia, and ether for maintainence after delivery of the infant. As experience was gained, side effects and complications became apparent. Ether and chloroform both relaxed the uterus, which was beneficial for intrauterine manipulation such as internal version and breech extraction, but caused uterine atony and postpartum haemorrhage. Ether in particular, with its sustained effect could lead to considerable haemorrhage. Both ether and chloroform caused pernicious post-operative nausea and vomiting in many patients. Chloroform was associated with rare cardiac deaths – later shown to be due to ventricular fibrillation. To a degree these complications could be minimised by the skill and experience of the anaesthetist – but skilled practitioners of anaesthesia were in short supply. As a result many surgeons and obstetricians preferred to operate without anaesthesia to avoid the rare but sometimes fatal complications. For example, in 1863, Horatio Storer, a professor of obstetrics in Boston, wrote *'In ordinary surgical practice it would be viewed as cruel, if not decidedly wrong, to perform an operation without the previous induction of anaesthesia. This, however, is as yet often considered unsafe, unnecessary or inadvisable in obstetric practice.....'* [22]

Munro Kerr, in the first edition of his classic text, Operative Midwifery, in 1908 pointed out an unusual problem associated with chloroform anaesthesia in hospitals lit by gas.[23]

'To some degree the frequency of bronchitis after caesarean section in my patients in the Glasgow Maternity Hospital may be accounted for by the fact that the operating-theatre is lit by gas, which, as has been frequently pointed out, decomposes the chloroform, setting free chlorine gas, which has a most irritating effect upon the bronchial mucous membrane.'

In the early 20th century anaesthetists administered ether and chloroform by dropping the solution onto a gauze mask held over the face; with no idea of the dose given and with only observation of respiration, pupils and the eyelid reflex to assess the depth of anaesthesia. However, the first half of the 20th century saw rapid developments in the safety of general anaesthesia. Anaesthetic machines held the compressed gases in cylinders with flow-control valves and vapourising bottles for ether and chloroform. The airway was controlled by endotracheal intubation. Induction of anaesthesia was greatly simplified in the 1930s by the use of short-acting intravenous barbiturates (Thiopental). The introduction of muscle relaxants (curare) in the 1940s completed the components needed to provide the modern era of so-called *'balanced anaesthesia.'* [17] Balanced anaesthesia was induced by intravenous thiopental and maintained by nitrous oxide, pain relief was supplemented with intravenous narcotics, muscle relaxants allowed control of the airway via endotracheal intubation and a relaxed abdominal wall for surgery. This became the standard of general anaesthetic care and remains so with newer induction drugs and inhalation agents, along with improved monitoring devices.

By the mid 20th century the particular vulnerability of the pregnant woman to regurgitation of highly acidic gastric juices, producing acid-aspiration (Mendelson's syndrome) while under general anaesthesia, was recognised.[19,24] The Confidential Enquiries into Maternal Deaths in England and Wales highlighted this as one of the main contributors to anaesthetic deaths and responsible for about 5% of all direct maternal mortality.[25] This served to emphasise the need for secure endotracheal intubation at all caesarean sections under general anaesthesia and helped provide impetus for the development of subspecialty obstetric anaesthetists. It also promoted the role of regional anaesthesia as an alternative to general anaesthesia for caesarean section.

Local anaesthesia

On 11th September, 1884, Carl Koller (1857-1944), an ophthalmologist in training at Vienna and working in conjunction with Sigmund Freud, discovered the local anaesthetic properties of cocaine on the eye.[26] This led to its use by injection for local infiltration and for regional nerve block anaesthesia. Koller was just applying to eye surgery what was already known – the numbing effect on the tongue of those who chewed the leaves of the coca plant, *Erythroxylon coca*. Many South Americans had been doing this to combat fatigue and hunger since the 1500s. The active principle, an alkaloid, had been isolated by the German chemist Albert Niemann and named cocaine in 1860. The toxic effects - convulsions and cardiovascular collapse - were soon recognised and to some extent ameliorated by using reduced concentrations. The addictive properties became manifest in those surgeons who carried out research on themselves with repeated nerve blocks.[17] In 1905 procaine (novocaine) became the standard local anaesthetic, until the development of lidocaine (lignocaine, xylocaine) in 1943.

With the availability of a safe and effective local anaesthetic many obstetricians chose the local infiltration technique in an attempt to avoid the complications of the alternatives; general or spinal anaesthesia. One such advocate was McIntosh Marshall (1901-1954), an obstetrician at the

Liverpool Maternity Hospital who wrote extensively on caesarean section and did much to popularise the lower-segment operation. In his 1939 text on caesarean section he advised local infiltration anaesthesia with procaine supplemented, if necessary, with inhalation of nitrous oxide at the most painful points of the operation; usually at delivery of the fetal head and closure of the peritoneum. He acknowledged that the technique required patience, *'A little less hurry, a little more care and trouble.'* [27] The reward, he said, was:

'The surgeon who has used local anaesthesia can leave the theatre with an easy conscience and a quiet mind. His patient has not run the anaesthetic gauntlet – ether and haemorrhage on the one hand, the tragic risks of spinal anaesthesia on the other.....Only by the persistent use of local anaesthesia can the inevitable fatality be indefinitely deferred.' [27]

DeLee in Chicago and Frey in Zurich were among many other obstetricians of the early 20th century who advocated local anaesthesia augmented by limited inhalation analgesia.[27]

Regional anaesthesia

William Halstead (1852-1922) working in New York's Roosevelt Hospital, and later the founding professor of surgery at Johns Hopkins University, demonstrated the feasibility of regional nerve blockade by injecting cocaine around a major sensory nerve in 1885. During his research he and his colleagues became addicted to cocaine; some of them died but Halstead survived, although he required large maintenance doses of morphine for the rest of his very productive life.[28]

The first spinal (subarachnoid) block using cocaine was reported in 1898 by the German surgeon, August Bier (1861-1949), in Leipzig.[17]

Some of the early landmark developments of regional anaesthesia in obstetrics are outlined below:
- 1900. The Basel obstetrician, Oskar Kreis (1872-1958), gave spinal anaesthesia with cocaine to six women in labour.[19,29]
- 1909. Walter Stoeckel (1871-1961), an obstetrician in Marburg, Germany, was the first to give an epidural injection of local anaesthetic to a woman in labour. He used procaine and the route of injection was via the sacral hiatus. Despite the good result he did not persist with this technique.[19,30]
- 1931. Eugen Aburel (1899-1975), a Romanian obstetrician, was the first to record the method of continuous epidural analgesia in labour with cinchocaine using a soft, flexible silk catheter threaded through a needle into the epidural space.[19,31]

- 1944. Edward Tuohy (1908-1959), an anaesthetist working at the Mayo Clinic, developed his eponymous needle with a lateral opening that allowed directional guidance and placement of a ureteral catheter to facilitate continuous spinal or epidural anaesthesia.[19,32]

By the early 20th century spinal anaesthesia was being given for caesarean section. Its advantages, in contrast to ether and chloroform, were that it did not cause uterine muscle relaxation and atonic haemorrhage, there was less postoperative vomiting and respiratory complications, and it did not lead to neonatal depression. However, with increasing experience, the peculiar susceptibility of the pregnant woman to sudden, profound and sometimes fatal cardiovascular collapse following spinal anaesthesia became apparent. This was such a catastrophic event that many obstetricians refused to use the technique. McIntosh Marshall, referred to previously as a champion of local anaesthesia, reviewed his own and others experience with spinal anaesthesia in the 1930s and had this to say[27]: '*.....experience leaves me in no doubt that spinal anaesthesia is particularly dangerous in caesarean section.*' He concluded his opinion with this chilling statement: '*Any obstetrician who sets out to perform a large series of caesarean sections under spinal anaesthesia must be prepared to face a possible mortality of not less than 1 per cent due to this cause alone.*' [27]

The problem was lack of knowledge about the local anaesthetic sympathetic blockade leading to profound hypotension and peripheral vasodilatation producing a functional hypovolaemia, compounded by aorto-caval compression in the supine position. By the mid 20th century physiological changes in the pregnant woman, along with the feto-placental circulatory interaction, were better understood. Preloading the intravascular space with crystalloid and knowledge of the supine hypotensive syndrome helped minimise the risk of significant hypotension. Epidural technique developed such that the midlumbar site was chosen as optimum to allow anaesthesia for both labour and caesarean delivery. Local anaesthetics improved and the longer acting bupivicaine became available in the late 1960s. The addition of opioids to the epidural or spinal infusion allowed a further reduction in the dose of local anaesthetic. Unless epidural anaesthesia was already in place for pain relief in labour the preferred technique for caesarean section was spinal anaesthesia. Smaller spinal needles reduced the risk of the previously troublesome incidence of postdural puncture headache.

The increasing complexity of available techniques and the understanding of the interrelationship between the fetus and mother inevitably led to the development of obstetric anaesthesia as a subspecialty in the latter part of the 20th century. This was aided by maternal mortality reviews which highlighted the significant contribution of substandard anaesthesia to maternal deaths associated with caesarean delivery. By the 21st century the availability of high standard obstetric anaesthesia enhanced the safety of caesarean delivery in well resourced hospitals, and substandard anaesthesia as a contributor to maternal deaths was greatly reduced.[33]

REFERENCES

1. Velpeau AL. An Elementary Treatise on Midwifery. Translated from the French by CD Meigs. Philadelphia: John Rigg; 1831. p516-7.
2. Astruc J. Elements of Midwifery. Translated by S. Ryley. London: S. Crowder and J. Coote; 1766.p162.
3. Blundell J. Lectures on the Principles and Practice of Midwifery. London: J. Masters;1839.p367.
4. Bergman NA. The Genesis of Surgical Anesthesia. Park Ridge: Wood Library-Museum of Anesthesiology; 1998. p18-19, 349-60.
5. Hamilton GR, Baskett TF. Mandrake to morphine: anodynes of antiquity. Ann R Coll Phys Surg Can 1999; 32:403-6.
6. Giuffra V. Surgical pain management at the Medical School of Salerno (11th-13th centuries). Vesalius 2013;19:3-6.
7. Infusino M, O'Neill S, Calmes S. Hog beans, poppies and mandrake leaves: a test of the efficacy of the Medieval soporific sponge. In: Atkinson RS, Boulton TB. (eds). The History of Anaesthesia. London: Parthenon Publishing Group; 1989. p29-33.
8. Hamilton GR, Baskett TF. In the arms of Morpheus: the development of morphine for postoperative pain relief. Can J Anesth 2000; 47:367-74.
9. Baker D, Cazalaa JB, Carli P. Larrey and Percy – a tale of two Barons. Resuscitation 2005;66:259-62.
10. Duncum BM. The Development of Inhalation Anaesthesia. London: Oxford University Press; 1947. p39, 499.
11. Shephard D. From Craft to Specialty: A Medical and Social History of Anesthesia. Thunder Bay, Ontario: York Point Publishing; 2009. p93.
12. Playfair WS. A Treatise on the Science and Practice of Midwifery. London: Smith, Elder and Co;1876. Vol 2, p222.
13. Radford T. On the Caesarean Section, Craniotomy, and Other Obstetric Operations. London: J&A Churchill; 1880. p37.
14. Simpson JY. Notes on the employment of sulphuric ether in the practice of midwifery. Monthly J Med Sci 1847;7:638-40.
15. Baskett TF. Edinburgh connections in a painful world. JR Coll Surg Edin Irel 2005;3:99-107.
16. Simpson JY. Discovery of a new anaesthetic agent, more effective than sulphuric ether. Lond Med Gazette 1847;40:934-7.
17. Sykes K, Bunker J. Anaesthesia and the Practice of Medicine: Historical

Perspectives. London: RSM Press; 2007. p25-32.
18. Davy H. Researches, Chemical and Philosophical: Chiefly Concerning Nitrous Oxide or Dephlogisticated Nitrous Air, and its Respiration. London: J. Johnson; 1800.
19. Baskett TF. On the Shoulders of Giants: Eponyms and Names in Obstetrics and Gynaecology. 2nd Edition, Cambridge: Cambridge University Press; 2008.
20. Klikovich S. Uber das stickstoffoxydul als anaestheticum bei geburten. Arch Gynakol 1881;18:81-108.
21. Spencer HR. Caesaren Section: With a Table of 120 Cases. London: John Bale, Sons and Danielson Ltd; 1925.p29-31.
22. Storer HR. On the employment of anaesthetics in obstetric medicine and surgery. Boston Med Surg J 1863;69:249-58.
23. Kerr JM. Operative Midwifery. London: Ballière, Tindall and Cox; 1908. p407.
24. Mendelson CL. The aspiration of stomach contents into the lungs during obstetric anesthesia. Am J Obstet Gynecol 1946; 52:191-205.
25. Report on Confidential Enquiries into Maternal Deaths in England and Wales, 1964-1966. London: HMSO; 1969. p68-75
26. Koller C. On the use of cocaine for producing anaesthesia on the eye. Lancet 1884;2:990-2.
27. Marshall CM. Caesarean Section: Lower Segment Operation. Bristol: John Wright and Sons Ltd; 1939. p57-80.
28. Nuland SB. Doctors: The Biography of Medicine. New York: Vintage Books;1989. p386-421.
29. Schreider MC, Holzgreve W. Oskar Kreis, a pioneer in spinal obstetric analgesia at the University Womens Clinic of Basel. Anaesthetist 2001;50:525-8.
30. Stoeckel IW. Uber sakrale anaesthesie. Zentrabl Gynakol 1909;33:1-15.
31. Aburel E. L'anesthesia locale continue (prolongée) en obstetrique. Bull Soc Obstet Gynec Paris. 1931;20:35-7.
32. Tuohy EB. Continuous spinal anesthesia: its usefulness and technique involved. Anesthesiology 1944;5:142-8.
33. Confidential Enquiry into Maternal Deaths in the United Kingdom. Why Mothers Die, 2000-2002. London: RCOG Press;2004. p122-134.

Chapter 14

Modern era of caesarean birth

For the *'modern era'* I have chosen the time period from the middle of the 20th century onward. To some extent this was an arbitrary choice, but it followed the Second World War and the considerable social and medical developments that ensued. This era saw great expansion in the use of caesarean delivery and an exponential increase in the safety of the operation. By the middle of the 20th century the main causes of maternal morbidity and mortality associated with caesarean delivery were: anaesthesia, haemorrhage, sepsis, ileus and thromboembolism.

Factors that increased the safety of caesarean delivery

- General improvement in socio-economic conditions, leading to a healthier population. This was enhanced by the development of national health services in many developed countries. Improved education and the availability of contraception led to a decrease in family size.
- Antenatal care organised along public health principles, including the treatment and prevention of anaemia.
- Organisation of regional and national audits of maternity outcomes. One of the best and most comprehensive of these was *The Confidential Enquiries into Maternal Deaths in England and Wales* – started in 1952, reporting every three years, and expanded in 1985 to include the whole United Kingdom.[1] These reports reviewed and highlighted the main causes of maternal death, and included detailed analysis of caesarean-related deaths with recommendations for improvement.
- Better perioperative care in the form of intravenous fluids and electrolyte balance.
- Improved anaesthesia services (see chapter 13).

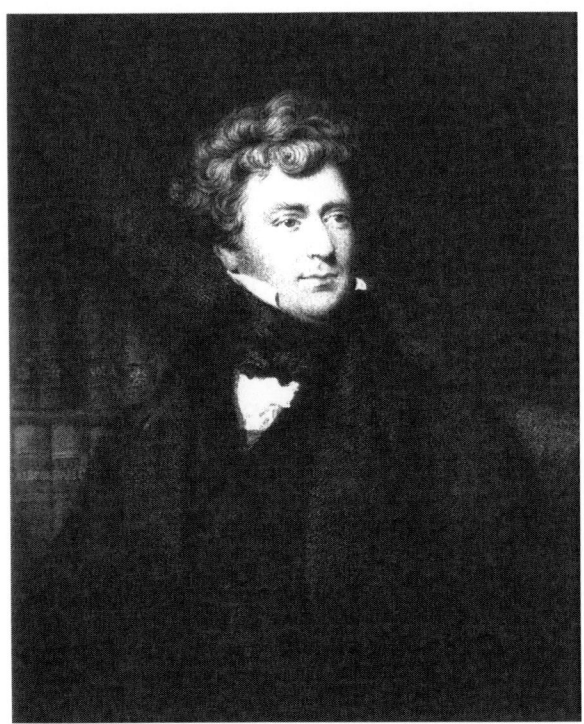

Figure 14.1
James Blundell (1790-1878)
Gave the first human-to-human blood transfusion in 1825. Through his surgical experiments with animals Blundell contributed much to the development of caesarean section, caesarean hysterectomy and tubal ligation. Criticised for his work on live animals he responded: 'Strike gentlemen, but hear... which will you sacrifice, your women or your cats?'

- Blood transfusion. The first successful human-to-human transfusion of blood was carried out by James Blundell of London in 1825 for a woman with postpartum haemorrhage.[2] (Figure 14.1) The ABO blood group system was established by Karl Landsteiner (1868-1943) of Vienna in 1901 and, along with Alexander Wiener (1907-1976) of New York, he discovered the Rhesus factor in 1940.[3,4] The next critical advance came from Richard Lewinshon (1895-1961) a surgeon in New York, but originally a medical graduate of Kiel University, Germany. In 1915, he made it feasible to store donated blood by adding the anticoagulant, 0.2% sodium citrate.[5] Blood transfusion was carried out to a limited degree following the First World War and by the 1940s regional and national blood banks were in place.[6]

- Uterotonic (oxytocic) drugs. Caesarean section was often done after a prolonged labour and, in such cases, the exhausted uterus was prone to relax leading to atonic haemorrhage. The first effective injectable oxytocic drug, ergometrine (ergonovine), was developed in 1935 – based on the previous observations that powdered ergot caused strong uterine contractions. At approximately twenty year epochs further oxytocic drugs were developed: oxytocin (1950s), 15-methyl prostaglandin F2 alpha (1970s) and misoprostol (1990s)[7,8] These agents dramatically reduced the risk of postpartum haemorrhage.
- Antibacterial drugs. The potential impact of these agents is seen in one of the first population–based reviews of maternal mortality in New York from 1930 to 1932. The main cause of death was infection, which was responsible for 49% of all caesarean–related deaths.[9] The first antibacterial agent, Prontosil (sulphanilamide), was developed in 1935 and was active against streptococci- one of the main causes of intrapartum sepsis. Other sulphonamides were produced, followed by penicillin in 1941 and streptomycin in 1944. Broad spectrum antibiotics followed: tetracycline, ampicillin and the cephalosporins among others. The first trial of chemoprophylaxis against infection during labour was by Harry Mayes of Brooklyn, New York in 1925.[10] He used 2% mercurochrome solution instilled into the vagina at each examination, and reduced the sepsis-related caesarean mortality.[10,11] Antibiotic prophylaxis was first used in caesarean section by Miller and Crichton of South Africa in 1968.[12] They gave ampicillin pre and postoperatively and reduced the infectious morbidity. By the 1980s the use of prophylactic broad spectrum antibiotics, usually a single intravenous dose, was widely accepted and later endorsed by Cochrane evidence-based reviews.[13]
- Thromboprophylaxis. In the 1950s, Sir Andrew Claye (1896-1976), Professor of Obstetrics at Leeds University and later President of the Royal College of Obstetricians and Gynaecologists, drew attention to the fact that the risk of fatal pulmonary embolism was six times higher following caesarean compared to vaginal delivery.[14] The contribution of enforced *'confinement'* to bed after caesarean section to the development of deep vein thrombosis was slowly recognised. Even in the early 20th century women were confined to bed for 7-14 days after delivery, in the belief that this would reduce the risk of subsequent utero-vaginal prolapse. Sometimes their legs were tied together to *'prevent infection'*. Early ambulation after delivery was tried sporadically in the late 19th/early 20th centuries, mostly in Germany.[15] The Blitz in Second World War London provided the

incentive for an enforced trial of early postpartum ambulation. Women were encouraged to get out of bed from the first postpartum day so they could, if needed, walk to the air-raid shelters. With this practice a reduction in postpartum deep vein thrombosis was observed.[15] The anticoagulants, heparin (1937) and warfarin (1941) were increasingly used to treat deep vein thrombosis. By the 1980s pulmonary embolism was the most common reason for direct maternal death in the developed world, as the other main causes: haemorrhage, sepsis and eclampsia were reduced. In 1995 the Royal College of Obstetricians and Gynaecologists (RCOG) produced guidelines advising heparin prophylaxis for all caesarean deliveries, other than those without risk factors.[16] These guidelines were adopted nationally and in the next triennial maternal mortality review the number of deaths due to thromboembolism after caesarean section fell from fifteen to four.[17]

Further development of the surgical technique

- *Low transverse uterine segment incision*

The biggest advance was the slow, but ultimately complete acceptance of the lower segment caesarean section (see chapter 11). Furthermore, by the 1950s the low transverse incision was preferred to the low vertical. In comparison to classical caesarean section the maternal morbidity and mortality in cases of prolonged labour was greatly reduced. As a result the obstetrician could undertake a trial of labour, and even a trial of instrumental assisted vaginal delivery, knowing that even if caesarean delivery was ultimately needed it would carry low maternal risk. Not only was maternal morbidity and mortality reduced with the lower segment operation, but compared to the classical incision the uterine scar was ten times less likely to rupture in a subsequent pregnancy – paving the way for vaginal birth after previous caesarean (VBAC). In the modern era some 97% of all caesarean operations are of the low transverse type, with the low vertical and classical procedures used only if there is no access to the lower uterine segment (scarring, fibroids, placenta accreta) or if it is undeveloped, as in cases of extreme prematurity.

- *Delivery of the placenta*

Randomised trials have shown that manual removal of the placenta, compared to its delivery by controlled cord traction, increases blood loss, endometritis and hospital stay.[18]

- *Suture materials*

As we have seen in chapter 9, plain catgut was used in the 1800s but was of limited success in closing the thick upper uterine segment of the classical incision. By the late 1800s, as part of Lister's principles, catgut was treated with 5% chromic acid and the resultant 'chromic catgut' became the standard suture for closure of the uterine incision. In the 1960s new synthetic absorbable polymers were developed, so that by the 1970s/80s two of these, polyglycolic acid (Dexon) and polyglactin (Vicryl), began to replace chromic catgut in many but not all hospitals.[19]

- *Single versus double-layer closure of the uterine incision*

Since Munro Kerr established the role of the transverse lower segment incision the myometrium has been closed in two layers. In the 1990s some surgeons began to use single layer closure and this resulted in the saving of about seven minutes operating time and a slight reduction in blood loss.[20] However, one large cohort study showed a four-fold increase of uterine rupture in subsequent pregnancy for single compared to double-layer closure.[21] There is still inadequate data on the integrity of single versus double-layer myometrial scars in subsequent pregnancy and labour.

- *Closure versus non-closure of the peritoneum*

The recent trend to omit the closure of the visceral and parietal peritoneum has been supported by randomised trials showing reduced operating time and less postoperative pain with non-closure.[22] The long term effect on adhesion formation and fertility has not been adequately studied; although a recent report showed an increase in adhesions with non-closure.[23]

- *Misgav Ladach technique*

This technique was developed by Michael Stark at the Misgav Ladach Hospital in Jerusalem and named after that hospital.[24] The idea was to simplify all steps of the operation. In brief, the Joel Cohen transverse abdominal incision is used, which is about 2-3cm higher that the Pfannenstiel incision; the rectus sheath is opened at this higher level and the rectus muscles pulled apart with the fingers; the parietal peritoneum is stretched and entered bluntly with the index finger; the lower uterine segment peritoneum and muscle are divided transversely in the standard manner. After delivery of the baby and placenta, the uterine incision is closed in a single layer, the peritoneal layers are not closed, but the rectus sheath and skin are.[24] Compared to the standard lower segment technique through the Pfannenstiel incision the Misgav Ladach procedure has been shown to have a shorter operative duration and less blood loss, as well as reduced postoperative pain, fever and a shorter hospital stay.[25,26] The long term effects on adhesion formation, fertility and uterine scar integrity in subsequent pregnancy await further study.

Expanding indications for caesarean section

By the 1960s the maternal mortality with caesarean section had dropped to less than one percent, and in most countries with developed health services to 1 in 1000 or less. Obstetrics began to change from a clinical art to an increasingly scientific specialty. As the security of maternal survival was assured, obstetricians turned to the welfare of the second patient under their care – the fetus. In this they were aided by the increasing sophistication of methods available to assess the in utero health of the fetus: amniocentesis, fetal heart rate (FHR) monitors and ultrasound. The era of the fetus as a patient, rather than a passive bystander in pregnancy and labour, developed. This was especially so in the 1970s with the advent of real-time ultrasound, which provided a window to the fetus and its intrauterine environment. As a result, gestational age, fetal growth, structural anomalies and biophysical activities reflective of fetal oxygenation could be assessed in the antenatal period. FHR monitoring in labour could, to a degree, assess the level of fetal oxygenation during the stress of uterine contractions.

With the development of neonatology as a subspecialty of paediatrics in the 1960s/70s, it became apparent that three things threatened the integrity of the fetal brain during labour: infection, hypoxia and trauma. Thus, the focus of the midwife or obstetrician in labour became protection of the fetus, particularly the fetal brain. There was less tolerance of prolonged labour with infection, attempts were made to identify fetal hypoxia and to avoid potentially traumatic delivery. As a result the following categories of potential fetal or neonatal jeopardy became reasons for caesarean delivery:

- Antepartum fetal assessment suggesting marginal placental function, inadequate to withstand the stress of labour.
- Maternal disease: Selected cases of severe pre-eclampsia/ eclampsia, chronic hypertension, diabetes, morbid obesity, chronic renal disease and others.
- Antepartum haemorrhage: virtually all cases of placenta praevia and selected cases of abruptio placentae.
- Fetal 'distress' in labour became an increasingly common indication for caesarean section with the widespread application of intrapartum FHR monitoring in the 1970s/80s. The problem was, and is, that the interpretation of FHR monitor patterns is an inexact science, so its use resulted in an increase in caesarean section rates without a concomitant improvement in perinatal outcome.[27]
- Dystocia became the commonest reason for caesarean section in the nulliparous woman. This included cases of cephalo-pelvic disproportion, but the majority were for so-called 'non-progressive labour' and defied precise classification. Dystocia was almost always in the nulliparous and often older parturient. Robert Roy, a Canadian obstetrician, has put forward a Darwinian explanation for the frequent occurrence of dystocia in modern obstetrics.[28] He postulates that the advent of agriculture-based societies and their diet, compared to hunter-gatherers, led to smaller babies and therefore a slight reduction in pelvic size over thousands of years. As a result when the modern diet led to larger babies, the problem of dystocia arose. Both Roy and Gebbie cite the very low dystocia rates in the rare existing populations of hunter-gatherers.[28,29] One such group, the Canadian Inuit, in a population-based study carried out in the 1970s had a caesarean section rate of 1.6%, five-fold less than the rest of the province; dystocia occurred in only four of the 622 deliveries.[30] Others have supported this hypothesis.[31]
- Difficult assisted vaginal delivery was abandoned. In the 1950s high forceps delivery was discontinued, and by the early 2000s many obstetricians had given up assisted mid pelvis deliveries with forceps or vacuum.
- Breech delivery. Up to the 1960s the apocryphal aphorism, *'Show me a man delivering a breech and I will give you his obstetric worth,'*

reflected the emphasis put on skilled operative vaginal delivery as a measure of an obstetrician's competence. However, in the 1980s/90s, because of the perinatal risks associated with breech vaginal delivery, an increasing number of obstetricians chose to deliver most, and sometimes all breeches by caesarean section. By the end of the 20th century most obstetricians, where safe caesarean facilities existed, were *'voting with their scalpels.'* Their bias was confirmed in 2000, with publication of the international term breech randomised-controlled trial, which showed a reduction in perinatal death and serious neonatal morbidity in those delivered by caesarean section.[32] The merits of the trial have been disputed by some, but even those who advocate the retention of breech vaginal delivery use caesarean section in 78%[33] to 90%[34] of cases. The detailed aspects of this debate are beyond the scope of this book, but have been covered elsewhere.[35,36]

- Other malpresentations, such as brow, face and transverse lie are now virtually all delivered by caesarean section.
- Twins. The approach to twin delivery has been comparable to that of the breech – a reluctance to accept even the slight increased risk of vaginal delivery. However, the recent international randomised trial, the Twin Birth Study, has confirmed that in experienced hands vaginal delivery of twins is as safe as caesarean section.[37] Nonetheless, the caesarean delivery rate for twins continues to rise and is 50-75% in many hospitals.
- Repeat caesarean section. As the primary caesarean delivery rate rose, so too did the repeat caesarean rate – which is now the commonest indication for caesarean section in many regions.

The indications for caesarean section vary from country to country and from hospital to hospital, but the big four indications account for 70-90% of all caesarean sections:

1. repeat caesarean section (35-40%)
2. dystocia (20-35%)
3. breech (10-15%)
4. fetal distress (10-15%)

In many cases it is not a clear-cut single indication, but a combination of dystocia and fetal distress in a non-progressive labour with a non-reassuring or suspicious FHR pattern.

In the last fifteen years the 10-group classification system of caesarean section developed by Michael Robson has been applied in many countries and hospitals.[38] This consistently shows that the biggest contributor to the caesarean section rate is dystocia in the nulliparous woman at term, with a single, cephalic fetus – either with spontaneous or induced labour.[39] Dystocia is responsible for almost half of all primary caesarean sections, most of which are in nulliparous woman destined to have a repeat caesarean delivery. Thus, directly or indirectly, dystocia is responsible for about two-thirds of all caesarean deliveries.

Most of the above discussion applies to developed countries with relatively sophisticated health services. In developing countries (where 80% of children are born) the main indications for caesarean delivery are cephalo-pelvic disproportion (CPD) and repeat caesarean section.[40] While dystocia and CPD are similar indications, the presentation in developing countries is quite different. The CPD cases follow prolonged, sometimes neglected, obstructed labour with the mother exhausted, dehydrated and infected. Uterine rupture occurs in about 10%, and is one of the leading causes of direct maternal death.[40]

Changing obstetric practice

The increased use of induction of labour and epidural analgesia in labour have both been implicated as contributing to the rising caesarean rates.[41,42] Greater use of both induction and epidural occurred in parallel with the increasing caesarean rates in the late 20th/early 21st century – but cause and effect are unproven.

The widespread use of electronic FHR monitoring, even for low risk pregnancy, can be a contributing factor – as noted above.[27]

The reduced use of operative vaginal delivery has led to generations of trainees with limited or no experience in these procedures, so that their perceived lack of safety has become a self-fulfilling prophecy.

Changing maternal demographics

This is a much more important factor than is usually acknowledged. The age of the obstetric population, particularly primigravidas, has increased steadily over the past 30-40 years.[43,44] This also applies to maternal obesity levels which have risen remarkably over the same time. In addition, older and overweight women have more co-morbidities – particularly hypertension and diabetes. Maternal weight gain in pregnancy and the weight of their babies have also increased significantly.[43,44] The parity spectrum has changed dramatically, so that instead of nulliparous women making up 20-25% of the obstetric population, they now constitute close to 50%. Dystocia is the commonest reason for primary caesarean section and this occurs almost exclusively in the nulliparous patient. Ineffective uterine action in labour, culminating in dystocia, is more common in the older gravida and in the obese.[43,44] Thus, in one generation, we have a greatly changed obstetric population; to an older, obese, more nulliparous group with more co-morbidities and bigger babies – one that is set up for higher rates of non-progressive, dystocic labour, leading to caesarean section.

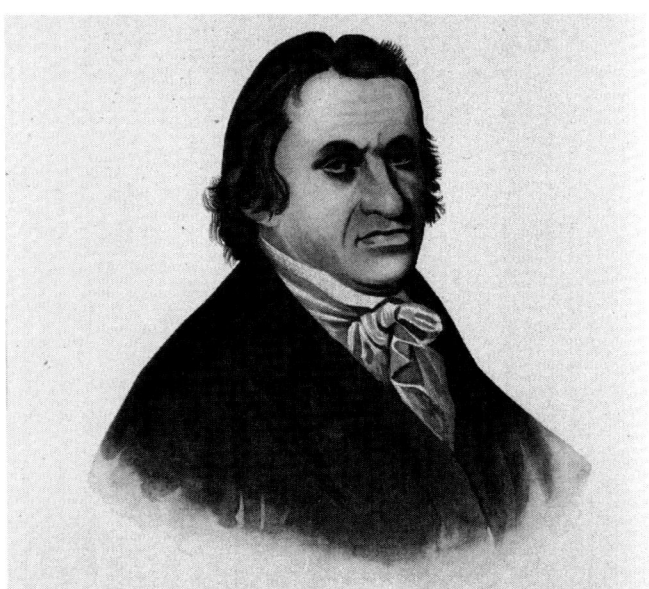

Figure 14.2
Samuel Bard (1742-1821)
Two hundred years ago he noted the three characteristics of pregnant women that predispose to dystocia: nulliparity, increased maternal age and obesity.

It should be noted, in the *'There is nothing new under the sun'* category, that similar observations were made by Samuel Bard of New York more than two hundred years ago. (Figure 14.2) In the section of his 1807 book, entitled *'Tedious and Difficult Labours'* he described the maternal characteristics that can lead to dystocia:[45]

'First child…..in some measure it may be said to be natural, and therefore necessary, for women with their first child…..to have more tedious labours than with those which follow…..

The same delay happens more certainly, and in a greater degree, when women are advanced beyond thirty years of age before they have a child…..

Very fat women are observed to be subject to slow labours, from a remarkably feeble action of the womb.'

Today we have a greater proportion of the obstetric population in all three categories.

Changing societal expectations

From the late 20th century parents came to expect the perfect outcome to every pregnancy, and to some extent this view was encouraged by the medical and midwifery establishment. If there was a poor outcome, many parents felt there must have been substandard practice at some point within the system. In truth, there are cases of substandard care that lead to injury, usually to the infant, and many of these involve delay or failure to perform caesarean section. Even though such cases are rare, they usually involve serious infant disability (cerebral palsy), and therefore the financial settlements are large. From the 1980s, earlier in the USA, but ultimately spreading to all developed countries, obstetrics became the most costly medical litigation specialty. As a result obstetricians began to carry out litigation–defence in their clinical practice. This often involved borderline cases, such as non-reassuring FHR patterns, breech presentation and the need for assisted mid pelvis delivery. The easier, and is some cases the more prudent decision was to move to caesarean section, rather than persist with attempts to achieve vaginal delivery. It should be pointed out that good clinical practice, with awareness of potential perinatal compromise, and litigation defensive medicine are, to a degree, one and the same.

The details of informed consent became more important and patients' aversion to risk increased. This was addressed in an Australian study of patients' and staff thresholds of clinical risk.[46] Some 600 women in late pregnancy and 294 staff (obstetricians, trainees and midwives) were asked what level of serious perinatal harm (death or lifelong disability) would they be willing to accept to avoid caesarean section and achieve vaginal birth. For 22% of women, a risk of 1 in 10,000 was too high and for 54.6% a risk of 1 in 1000 was unacceptable.[46] For the staff, 50% found the risk of 1 in 1000 too high. It is difficult to provide precise levels of risk for obstetric procedures, but for many patients (and even staff) their risk threshold would be exceeded by the fetal and neonatal risks of assisted vaginal delivery, malpresentations and vaginal birth after a caesarean (VBAC).

Caesarean section rates

In the developed world caesarean section rates rose slowly through the first part of the 20th century to reach 3-6% by 1970. In the 1970s the changing attitude to the fetus as a patient, along with development of neonatal intensive care, caused a rapid rise in the use of caesarean section. In addition, for reasons outlined earlier in this chapter, the caesarean-related maternal mortality fell to less than 1 in 1000. For example, in England and Wales, the caesarean maternal death rate fell from 3.3/1000 in 1957 to 0.8/1000 in 1977.[47]

The plethora of published caesarean section rates can be overwhelming, and they are accessible.[48-55] Some examples are shown below:

Australia	1985 (16%) → 2011 (32%)
Canada	1970 (6%) → 2014 (27.5%)
England & Wales	1957 (2.4%) → 2000 (21.5%)
France	1972 (6.1%) → 2008 (18.8%)
Italy	1980 (11%) → 2008 (38%)
Netherlands	1968 (3.5%) → 2010 (16.7%)
Nordic countries (Finland, Norway, Sweden, Denmark)	1970 (2-6%) → 2008 (16-21%)
United Kingdom	2008 (22%) → 2013 (26.2%)
United States	1970 (6%) → 2014 (32.2%)

A World Health Organization (WHO) report of caesarean rates in 2008 included 137 countries, covering 95% of global births that year.[51] Fifty-four of the countries had caesarean section rates below 10%, the level at which the WHO found higher maternal and neonatal mortality rates (see later). Fourteen countries, mostly in Africa, had caesarean rates ≤ 2%.[51] The United States has long been cited as a country with a high caesarean section rate, but this study showed that eleven countries had higher rates than the USA (30.3%); ranging from Uruguay (31.8%) to Brazil (45.9%).[51] In addition to Brazil, two countries, Iran and the Dominican Republic, had caesarean rates > 40%.[51]

Another WHO study compared the change in caesarean rates from 1990 to 2014 in six global regions, comprising 121 countries.[52] There was a universal rise in rates, as follows:

Region	1990	2014
Africa	2.9	7.4
Asia	4.4	19.5
Europe	11.2	25.0
North America	22.3	32.3
Oceania	18.5	32.6
Latin America + Caribbean	22.8	42.2

(Rates are in per cent)

The range of caesarean section within the nineteen countries of one of these regions, Latin America, was 1.6% to 40.0% in a previous 1996-97 review.[49] In all regions, countries, hospitals, and within hospitals among individual obstetricians, caesarean section rates vary considerably. Another universal finding is higher rates in private obstetric units and among higher socio-economic groups.

In 1985 the WHO published a list of fifteen recommendations related to the application of perinatal technology in labour and delivery.[56] These were the result of a consensus conference held in April 1985 at Fortaleza, Brazil. Two of the recommendations applied to caesarean delivery:

- *'There is no justification in any specific geographic region to have more than 10 to 15% caesarean section births.*
- *There is no evidence that a caesarean section is required after a previous transverse low segment caesarean section birth. Vaginal delivery after caesarean should normally be encouraged whenever emergency surgical capacity is available.'* [56]

Following this there was some guilt and a certain amount of hand-wringing, as hospitals and regions tried to reduce or explain their higher caesarean section rates. However, despite the admonition of the WHO, there has been a global rise in the caesarean rate – in some countries to three or four fold higher than the WHO's advice. Commenting on the trend for academics and organisations to define 'ideal' caesarean section rates, Ronald Cyr systematically reviewed the many and varied factors that lead to the clinical decision to perform caesarean section. He concluded there could be no practical application of a theoretical ideal rate: *'The cesarean rate is, thus, a consequence of subjective clinical decisions, and cannot be preordained. An ideal cesarean rate cannot be defined outside of a framework of individual values and assumptions.'* [57] Robson also criticised the obsession with caesarean rates: *'Overall, caesarean section rates are unhelpful and should not be judged in isolation from other outcomes and epidemiological characteristics.'* [39] He also noted, *'Discussions about reducing caesarean section rates without taking other factors into account are, at best, inappropriate and, at worst, dangerous.'* [39]

In 2014 a WHO study group carried out a systematic review of published, worldwide, population-based studies and analyzed the relationship between caesarean section rates and maternal and neonatal mortality.[58] They found a decrease in mortality as caesarean rates rose to 10-15%. The critical rate was 10% - below which mortality was higher. But as the caesarean rate rose above 10%, and up to 30%, there was no further improvement in mortality.[58] This was challenged by another review of similar international data, which concluded there was continued improvement in maternal and neonatal death rates with caesarean section rates up to 19%.[59]

In the developed world, because the levels of maternal and neonatal mortality were so low, many practicing obstetricians felt this was no longer an adequate representation of the standard of care. Increasingly they turned to estimates of severe maternal, neonatal and infant morbidity, and their long-term implications, as the more relevant measure of clinical and medico-legal outcomes. Thus, notwithstanding the WHO pronouncements, caesarean section rates keep rising and will probably continue to do so as women choose to have fewer children at a later age.

Vaginal birth after caesarean section (VBAC)

'Once a caesarean always a caesarean' came to be known as *'Craigin's dictum,'* after Edwin Craigin (1859-1918), of New York, included this phrase in a lecture to the Eastern Medical Society of New York on 12 May 1916. This was published later that year:[60]

'One thing must always be borne in mind, viz, that no matter how carefully a uterine incision is sutured, we can never be certain that the cicatrized uterine wall will stand a subsequent pregnancy and labour without rupture. This means that the usual rule is, once a caesarean always a caesarean.'

Although Craigin is consistently cited as the first to declare this dictum, Cyr points out that others used the same phrase before Craigin, and it was probably already well established both in the United States and Europe.[61,62] When this dictum was proposed all caesarean sections were of the classical type and the indication in the vast majority of cases was contracted pelvis; so it made good obstetric sense. By the 1940s/50s the lower segment caesarean technique had largely replaced the classical caesarean section, thus lowering ten-fold the risk of scar rupture in a subsequent pregnancy and labour. In addition, the indications for caesarean delivery widened to include non-recurrent reasons. By the 1970s, in many countries, a majority of women with a previous lower segment caesarean underwent a trial for vaginal delivery in a subsequent pregnancy – with success rates of 50-80%. At this time VBAC was generally accepted as a safe option, although no less an authority than Sir Norman Jeffcoate of Liverpool sounded a cautious note in 1971.[63] Reviewing the risks of VBAC he and his Liverpool colleagues wrote:

'Although caesarean section is, in general, more dangerous than vaginal delivery, it is probably less dangerous (for both mother and baby) than is vaginal delivery from a uterus whose lower segment is scarred as the result of a previous section......the allowing of vaginal delivery, or attempted vaginal delivery, after previous caesarean section......should, perhaps, be the exception

rather than the rule.' [63]

The United States and Canada were slower to adopt VBAC, but by the 1980s national consensus conference statements, and the WHO as previously noted, promoted trial of vaginal delivery after previous caesarean, *'In hospitals with appropriate facilities, services, and staff for prompt emergency cesarean birth…..'* [64,65] National professional organisations encouraged medical and midwifery staff to offer VBAC to women with spontaneous labour and one previous uncomplicated transverse lower segment caesarean. As the rates of primary caesarean section increased worldwide, so too did the practice of VBAC. However, it was not long before the *'pendulum syndrome'* of obstetric care took over. Excessive zeal to achieve VBAC moved some to promote VBAC in cases with more than one previous caesarean, to induce and augment labour with oxytocic drugs, and to include complicated pregnancies, such as twins. With the increased number of VBAC attempts, and the inclusion of more complex cases, the rare episodes of uterine rupture emerged – with sometimes catastrophic clinical and litigation sequelae. Thus, by the 2000s the pendulum reversed direction and VBAC became a rare or non-existent event in many hospitals.

Much has been written on this subject and most obstetricians now follow various national guidelines, which define the personnel and facilities needed for this endeavour.[66-69] Informed consent, with realistic information on the perinatal risk in the event of uterine rupture, plays a major role in patient selection.[36,70] The dilemma facing those in low resource countries has also been reviewed.[71]

Sterilisation and caesarean section

Thomas Denman had a radical social proposal to prevent the recurrence of pregnancy in women *'…..so unfortunately framed, that she cannot have a living child.'* [72] He acknowledged that craniotomy was necessary to save the mother, but baulked at performing this repeatedly in the same woman. He therefore proposed, *'When it has been ascertained that women could not possibly bear living children and one great end of marriage has been frustrated, some have determined on a voluntary separation from their husbands, from a sense of the moral turpitude of conceiving children without the chance of bringing them living into the world …..many evils might thereby be prevented.'* [72]

Apart from caesarean hysterectomy some of the earlier surgeons carried out oophorectomy at the time of caesarean section to prevent future pregnancy. James Blundell was the first to propose the simpler and more humane approach of tubal ligation at the time of caesarean section: *'Before closing the abdomen, the operator, I conceive, ought to remove a portion, say one line, of the fallopian tube, right and left, so as to intercept its caliber......Mere division of the tube might be sufficient to produce sterility, but the further removal of a portion of the tube appears to be the surer practice....*'[73] The first to carry this out was SS Lungren of Toledo, Ohio in May 1880.[74] The patient was a woman who had childhood rickets causing a contracted pelvis. He had carried out a successful caesarean section in 1875 and at this, her second caesarean, also successful, '*.....the Fallopian tubes were tied instead with a strong silk ligature about one inch from their uterine attachment.*' [74] Multiple variations followed, including the development of simple tubal ligation procedures in the early 20th century by Madlener, Irving and Pomeroy – with the latter technique gaining widespread acceptance.[75] For a time in the mid 20th century caesarean hysterectomy was used for sterilisation purposes in some hospitals (see chapter 12).

In the late 19th/early 20th century obstetricians debated the pros and cons of sterilisation at the time of caesarean section and the degree of choice for the patient. John Whitridge Williams distinguished between '*pauper*' patients and women '*in the upper walks of life.*' [76] The '*former he advised*' to have a tubal ligation or hysterectomy with their first caesarean, as they might '*neglect to place themselves under proper surroundings for a subsequent operation.*' For the women in the '*upper walks of life*' he tried to dissuade them from sterilisation at the first caesarean, lest the infant die.[76] By the mid 20th century the principles of informed consent for sterilisation operations was entrenched.

Compelled caesarean delivery

The doctrine of informed consent is balanced by that of informed refusal, such that any patient has the right to refuse any medical or surgical treatment offered – however compelling the benefits of that treatment may be. A unique situation exists in obstetrics when the pregnant woman may refuse treatment on behalf of her fetus; so-called '*maternal-fetal conflict.*' The involved obstetrician therefore has to balance the obligation to respect maternal autonomy with the duty of beneficence to the fetus. In many cases the decision involves a medically indicated caesarean section for fetal reasons, although in cases such as complete placenta praevia benefit to the mother is also a consideration.

It is very rare for a woman to refuse a medically advised caesarean section if the reasons for the decision are carefully explained. Even if the woman was hoping for a vaginal delivery, she will nearly always forgo her own wishes and take on personal risk if she feels it will benefit her baby. Nonetheless, cases of competent, fully informed women refusing medically recommended caesarean section do occur and on very rare occasions court-ordered caesarean section has been carried out.[77,78] These were only considered when there was judged to be a high probability that the caesarean would be life-saving or prevent permanent damage to the fetus, and the additional risk to the mother was low.[70] One of the problems in these cases is that the clinical and technical appraisal of fetal health that leads to the decision for caesarean section is often uncertain and imprecise.[79] The current recommendations are against coercion or court-ordered interventions and in favour of complete respect for the woman's autonomy over both herself and her fetus.[70,80] Hospitals should formulate their own guidelines for these rare situations, giving consideration to local clinical, ethical and legal factors.

Posthumous caesarean delivery

When accident or catastrophic intracranial disease leads to brain death in pregnancy, the woman can sometimes be maintained on life support. In the second and third trimester consideration may be given to sustain the mother's somatic function to allow the fetus to mature sufficiently to be delivered by caesarean section. These instances of *'posthumous motherhood'* are rare, and a recent review collected only thirty cases between 1982 and 2010.[81] These present ethical and clinical challenges, and of the thirty cases, twelve viable infants were born and six were normal at two year follow up.[81]

REFERENCES

1. Report on Confidential Enquiries into Maternal Deaths in England and Wales, 1952-54. London: Her Majesty's Stationary Office; 1956.
2. Baskett TF. James Blundell: The first transfusion of human blood. Resuscitation 2002;52:229-33.
3. Figl M, Pelinka LE. Karl Landsteiner, the discoverer of blood groups. Resuscitation 2004;63:251-4.
4. Landsteiner K, Wiener AS. An agglutinable factor in human blood recognized by immune serum for rhesus blood. Proc Soc Exp Biol Med 1940;43:223-30.
5. Lewinshon R. Blood transfusion by the citrate method. Surg Gynecol Obstet 1915;21:37-47.
6. Giangrande PL. The history of blood transfusion. Br J Haematol 2000;110:758-67.
7. Baskett TF. The development of prostaglandins. Best Pract Res Clin Obstet

Gynaecol 2003;17:703-6.
8. Baskett TF. The development of oxytocic drugs in the management of postpartum haemorrhage. Ulster Med J 2004;73:2-6.
9. Hooker RS. Maternal Mortality in New York City: A Study of All Puerperal Deaths, 1930-1932. New York: Oxford University Press; 1933.
10. Mayes HW. The use of mercurochrome during labor. Am J Obstet Gynecol 1925;6:69-72.
11. Willson JR. The conquest of cesarean section-related infections: A progress report. Obstet Gynecol 1988;72:519-32.
12. Miller RD, Crichton D. Ampicillin prophylaxis in caesarean section. S Afr J Obstet Gynaecol 1968;6:69-72.
13. Gyte GM, Dou L, Vazquez JC. Different classes of antibiotics given to women routinely for preventing infections at caesarean section. Cochrane Database Syst Rev 2014:CD008726.
14. Claye A. Caesarean section – a lethal operation? J Obstet Gynaecol Br Commonw 1961;68:577-83.
15. Van Stralen KJ, Terveer EM, Doggan CJM, Helmerhorst FM, Vandenbroucke JP. The tortous history of the implementation of early ambulation after delivery. J R Soc Med 2007;100:90-6.
16. Report of the RCOG Working Party on Prophylaxis Against Thromboembolism in Gynaecology and Obstetrics. London: RCOG Press;1995.
17. The Confidential Enquiries into Maternal Deaths in the United Kingdom, 1997-1999. London: RCOG Press; 2001.
18. Anorlu R, Maholwana B, Hofmeyr GJ, Methods of delivering the placenta at caesarean section. Cochrane Database Syst Rev 2008: CD004737.
19. Muffly TM, Tizzano AP, Walters MD. The history and evolution of sutures in pelvic surgery. J R Soc Med 2011;104:107-112.
20. Dodd JM, Anderson ER, Gates S. Surgical techniques for uterine incision and uterine closure at the time of caesarean section. Cochrane Database Syst Rev 2008:CD004732.
21. Bujold E, Bujold C, Hamilton EF, Havel F, Gauthier R. The impact of single-layer or double-layer closure on uterine rupture. Am J Obstet Gynecol 2002;186:1326-30.
22. Bamigboye AA, Hofmeyr GJ. Closure versus non-closure of the peritoneum at caesarean section. Cochrane Database Syst Rev 2014:CD000163.
23. Lyell DJ, Caughey AB, Hu E, Daniels K. Peritoneal closure at primary cesarean delivery and adhesions. Obstet Gynecol 2005;106:275-80.
24. Holmgren G, Sjoholm L, Stark M. The Misgav Ladach method for cesarean section: method description. Acta Obstet Gynecol Scand 1999;78:615-21.
25. Darj E, Nordstrom ML. Misgav Ladach method for cesarean section compared to the Pfannenstiel method. Acta Obstet Gynecol Scand 1999;78:37-41.
26. Mathai M, Hofmeyr GJ, Mathai NE. Abdominal surgical incisions for caesarean section. Cochrane Database Syst Rev 2013: CD004453.
27. Alfirevic Z, Devane D, Gyte GML. Continuous cardiotocography (CTG) as

a form of electronic fetal monitoring (EFM) for fetal assessment during labour. Cochrane Database Syst Rev 2013:CD006066.
28. Roy RP. A Darwinian view of obstructed labour. Obstet Gynecol 2003;102:397-401.
29. Gebbie DAM. Reproductive Anthropology – Descent Through Woman. Chichester: John Wiley and Sons;1981.
30. Baskett TF. Obstetric care in the central Canadian Arctic. BMJ 1978;2:1001-4.
31. Liston WA. Rising caesarean section rates: can evolution and ecology explain some of the difficulties of modern childbirth? J R Soc Med 2003;96:559-61.
32. Hannah ME, Hannah WJ, Hewson SA ED, Saigal S, Willan AR. Planned caesarean section versus planned vaginal birth for breech presentation at term: a randomised multicentre trial. Lancet 2000;356:1375-83.
33. Goffinet F, Carayol M, Foidart JM et al. For the PREMODA Study Group. Is planned vaginal delivery for breech presentation at term still an option? Results of an observational survey in France and Belgium. Am J Obstet Gynecol 2006;194:1002-11.
34. Hehir MP, O'Connor HD, Kent EM et al. Changes in vaginal breech delivery rates in a single large metropolitan area. Am J Obstet Gynecol 2012;206:498-504.
35. Hofmeyr GT, Hannah M, Lowrie TA. Planned caesarean section for term breech delivery. Cochrane Database Syst Rev 2015: CD000166.
36. Baskett TF. Essential Management of Obstetric Emergencies. 5th edition. Bristol: Clinical Press Ltd;2015.
37. Barrett JFR, Hannah ME, Hutton EK et al. A randomized trial of planned cesarean or vaginal delivery for twin pregnancy. N Engl J Med 2013;369:1295-1305.
38. Robson M. Classification of caesarean sections. Fetal Matern Med Rev 2001;12:23-39.
39. Robson M, Hartigan L, Murphy M. Methods of achieving and maintaining an appropriate caesarean section rate. Best Pract Res Clin Obstet Gynaecol 2013;27:297-308.
40. Kwawukume EY. Caesarean section in developing countries. Best Pract Res Clin Obstet Gynaecol 2001;15:165-78.
41. Dunne C, DaSilva O, Schmidt G, Natale R. Outcomes of elective labour induction and elective caesarean section in low-risk pregnancies between 37 and 41 weeks gestation. J Obstet Gynaecol Can 2009;19:1124-30.
42. Schuit E, Kwee A, Westerhuis ME et al. A clinical prediction model to assess the risk of operative delivery, BJOG 2012;119:915-23.
43. Cnattinguis R, Cnattinguis S, Notzon FC. Obstacles to reducing cesarean rates in a low cesarean setting: the effect of maternal age, height and weight. Obstet Gynecol 1998;92:501-6.
44. Joseph KS, Young DC, Dodds L et al. Changes in maternal characteristics and obstetric practice and recent increases in primary cesarean delivery.

Obstet Gynecol 2003;102:791-800.
45. Bard S. A Compendium of the Theory and Practice of Midwifery. New York: Collins and Perkins; 1807.p134-6.
46. Walker SP, McCarthy EA, Ugoni A et al. Cesarean delivery or vaginal birth: A survey of patient and clinical thresholds. Obstet Gynecol 2007;109:67-72.
47. Reports on Confidential Enquiries into Maternal Deaths in England and Wales. 1964-1966;1970-1972;1976-1978. London: Her Majesty's Stationery Office; 1969, 1975 and 1982.
48. Notzon FC. International differences in the use of obstetric interventions. JAMA 1990;263:3286-3291.
49. Belizan JM, Althabe F, Barros FC, Alexander S. Rates and implications of caesarean sections in Latin America: ecological study. BMJ 1999;319:1397-1402.
50. The National Sentinel Caesarean Section Audit Report. London: Royal College of Obstetricians and Gynaecologists; 2001.
51. Gibbons L, Belizan JM, Lauer JA et al. The global numbers and costs of additionally needed and unnecessary caesarean sections performed per year: Overuse as a barrier to universal coverage. World Health Report Background Paper, No30. Geneva: World Health Organization; 2010.
52. Bretan AP, Ye J, Moller A et al. The increasing trend in caesarean section rates: global, regional and national estimates: 1990-2014. PLoS One 2016;11:e0148343.
53. Evaluation of Cesarean Delivery. Washington DC: American College of Obstetricians and Gynecologists;2001.
54. Li Z, Zeki R, Hilder L, Sullivan EA. Australia's mothers and babies 2011. Canberra: AIHW National Perinatal Epidemiology and Statistics Unit;2013.
55. Zhao Y, Zhang J, Hukkelhoven C et al. Modest rise in caesarean section from 2000-2010: The Dutch experience. PLos One 2016;11: e0155565.
56. World Health Organisation. Appropriate technology for birth. Lancet 1985;2:436-7.
57. Cyr RM. Myth of the ideal cesarean section rate: commentary and historic perspective. Am J Obstet Gynecol 2006;194:932-6.
58. WHO Statement on Caesarean Section Rates. Geneva: World Health Organization; 2015.
59. Molina G, Weiser TG, Lipsitz SR et al. Relationships between cesarean delivery rate and maternal and neonatal mortality. JAMA 2015;314:2263-70.
60. Craigin EB. Conservatism in obstetrics. NY Med J 1916;104:1-3.
61. Cyr RM. Historical Perspective: "Once a cesarean .....always a cesarean." ACOG Clin Review 2004;9:12-14. American College of Obstetricians and Gynecologists, Washington DC.
62. Green CM. Cesarean section: a consideration of indications, technique, and time of operating. Boston Med Surg J 1916;174:441-50.
63. Case BD, Corcoran R, Jeffcoate TNA, Randle GH. Caesarean section and its place in modern obstetric practice. J Obstet Gynaecol Br Cwlth 1971;78:203-14.

64. NIH Consensus Development Statement on Cesarean Birth: The Caesarean Birth Task Force. Obstet Gynecol 1981;57:537-45.
65. Indications for cesarean section: final statement of the panel of the National Conference on Aspects of Cesarean Birth. Can Med Assoc J 1986;134:1348-52.
66. Society of Obstetricians and Gynaecologists of Canada. Guidelines for vaginal birth after previous caesarean birth. Clinical Practice Guideline No.155.Ottawa: SOGC:2005.
67. Royal College of Obstetricians and Gynaecologists. Birth after previous Caesarean birth. Green-top Guideline No.45. London: RCOG:2007.
68. American College of Obstetricians and Gynecologists. Vaginal birth after previous cesarean delivery. Practice Bulletin No.115. Washington, DC:ACOG;2010.
69. Royal Australian and New Zealand College of Obstetricians and Gynaecologists. Planned vaginal birth after caesarean section (Trial of labour). C-Obs 38. Victoria: RANZCOG;2010.
70. Harris LH. Counselling women about choice. Best Pract Res Clin Obstet Gynaecol. 2001;15:93-107.
71. Wanyonyi S, Muriithi FG. Vaginal birth after caesarean section in low resource settings: the clinical and ethical dilemma. J Obstet Gynaecol Can 2015;37:922-26.
72. Denman T. An Introduction to the Practice of Midwifery. Volume 2. London: J. Johnston;1798.p241-2.
73. Blundell J. Principles and Practice of Obstetricy. London: E. Cox;1834.
74. Lungren SS. A case of cesarean section twice successfully performed on the same patient. Am J Obstet Dis Women Child 1881;14:78-94.
75. Baskett TF. On the Shoulders of Giants: Eponyms and Names in Obstetrics and Gynaecology. 2nd Edition. Cambridge: Cambridge University Press; 2008.
76. Young JH. Caesarean Section: the History and Development of the Operation from Earliest Times. London: HK Lewis & Co Ltd;1944.p235-244.
77. Adams SF, Mahowald MB, Gallagher J. Refusal of treatment during pregnancy. Clin Perinatol 2003;30:127-40.
78. Deshpande NA, Oxford CM. Management of pregnant patients who refuse medically indicated cesarean delivery. Rev Obstet Gynecol 2012;5:e 144-50.
79. Kolder VE, Gallagher J, Parsons MT. Court-ordered obstetrical interventions. N Engl J Med 1987;316:1192-5.
80. American College of Obstetricians and Gynecologists. Committee Opinion No.664. Refusal of medically recommended treatment during pregnancy. Washington DC: ACOG;2016
81. Esmaeilzadeh M, Dictus C, Kayvanpour E et al. One life ends, another begins: Management of a brain-dead pregnant mother – A systematic review. BMC Med 2010 Nov18;8:74.

Chapter 15

Caesarean birth by maternal choice

'*Normal women come to us demanding a cesarean delivery to avoid the agonies of childbirth. While none would grant them this request, it is well to remember that what is a fantasy today may be a fact tomorrow.*' [1]

These prophetic words were delivered to a symposium on *Operative Delivery vs. Spontaneous Delivery* at the New York Obstetrical Society in 1920 by Oliver Paul Humpstone, Professor of Obstetrics at Brooklyn, New York.[1] He began his lecture by expressing, '*Apprehension lest one be considered a dangerous radical rather than a sane progressive thinker...*' [1] In fact, Humpstone was not advocating caesarean section at the mother's request, but supporting the expanding medical indications for the operation. He also pointed out that caesarean section was, '*the easiest way for any primiparous women to have her baby; and it is the surest way of having a live baby.*' [1]

Some thirteen years earlier, Edward Reynolds, obstetrician at the Free Hospital for Women in Boston, advised elective caesarean section:

'*.....in an exceedingly small class of over civilized women in whom the natural powers of withstanding pain and muscular fatigue are abnormally deficient.*' [2]

Trolle cited two early cases of caesarean section by maternal choice.[3] The first caesarean section in Denmark was done at maternal request on 26th October, 1813, in the village of Hillerod, near Copenhagen. The woman in question, a thirty-six year old primigravida, lived on a farm and had been in labour for two days but the baby's head remained above the pelvic brim. The local doctor called in an army surgeon, Dr Schlegel, and they both agreed there were three options: no intervention, high forceps or caesarean section. The doctors advised forceps but the woman and her husband insisted on caesarean delivery. The operation was done in the home without analgesia. The mother recovered sufficiently to request a glass of aquavit and a cup of coffee (both refused), but succumbed to peritonitis two days later. The child survived.[3]

In 1904, at the Maternity Hospital in Copenhagen, a thirty year old woman with a contracted pelvis was at the end of her seventh pregnancy. All six of her previous infants had been stillborn following traumatic operative vaginal delivery. Showing good obstetrical judgment, she asked for and received an elective caesarean section and tubal ligation; both she and her child survived.[3]

One could go back to 1769 and claim that the first recorded caesarean section by maternal choice was done by a woman on herself in Jamaica, as recounted in chapter 4.

In October 1960, Sir Andrew Claye, a past president of the RCOG, delivered the William Hunter Memorial lecture to the Glasgow Obstetrical and Gynaecological Society; the focus of his talk was the lethal complications of caesarean section.[4] He concluded his lecture by quoting a statement written by an American pathologist, adding comments of his own which, fifty years later, can be seen as remarkably prescient:

'Only a morbid anatomist and pathologist of Dr Schwartz's eminence would have the delightful and logical temerity to write: 'It is best to be born at term by caesarean section before the onset of labour.' But why not? It has already been done sporadically. Modern caesarean section with local analgesia has a maternal mortality no greater than that of natural childbirth with its unforeseen complications and, there being no birth injury, the perinatal mortality is much less. And caesarean birth would be a sort of millennium for women: no more relaxed vaginal outlets and utero-vaginal prolapse, goodbye to torn and infected cervices and cancer of the cervix. And surgical technique marches on and on. So, one day, why not? But my 'natural childbirth' conscience pricks me nevertheless.' [4]

The modern phase of caesarean birth by maternal choice started in the 1990s when those who were said to be *'too posh to push'* sparked the controversy. One of the earliest editorials on the subject reviewed the fetal risks in labour and suggested that women should be allowed to consider these risks and opt for a *'prophylactic'* caesarean section at term.[5] Many studies, papers and opinions followed – along with gainful employment for ethicists. In fact, obstetricians in private practice have probably acceded to such maternal requests since the mid 20th century – albeit under pseudo indications. The label *'too posh to push'* oversimplifies the reasons women increasingly request elective caesarean section. The literature on the subject is extensive so only the broad aspects will be covered here. It applies mostly to the developed world and to some private clinics in developing countries.

Reasons women choose elective caesarean delivery

- Fear of pain. With the availability of epidural analgesia this should no longer be a drawback to labour, but in hospitals with an incomplete epidural service this can be a factor.

- Tocophobia is the term used for a morbid fear of labour and childbirth, and this may prompt some women to seek elective caesarean delivery. It can be linked to a past history of sexual abuse or rape; in others it may result from a previous painful labour and traumatic delivery.[6] A study from Sweden found about 10% of pregnant women suffered fear of childbirth and, even after counselling, this group had a three to six times higher rate of elective caesarean section.[7]
- Fear of pelvic floor damage: episiotomy/perineal tears with pain and dyspareunia. Longterm: utero-vaginal prolapse, urinary, flatal and faecal incontinence, sexual dysfunction. The pelvic floor sequelae of vaginal versus caesarean delivery have not been fully clarified, but labour and vaginal delivery, particularly if assisted with forceps or vacuum, increase the risk. Any gynaecologist with clinical experience knows this.
- Fear of damage to or death of the baby. There are studies which show that the risks of perinatal asphyxia and trauma at birth are reduced with elective caesarean section compared to vaginal delivery.[8-10] The problem is the lack of long-term comparative outcomes.
- Eliminate rare intrapartum emergencies, such as abruptio placentae and cord prolapse.
- Eliminate the unexplained stillbirths that occur between thirty-nine and forty-one weeks gestation. This is counterbalanced by a comparable increase in unexplained stillbirth in a subsequent pregnancy with a caesarean scar.[11]
- Control and convenience:
  - A scheduled caesarean section allows the woman to have the obstetrician of her choice.
  - It is easier for the husband or partner to be present
  - Organisation of care for other children.

Potential obstetric and infant sequelae of elective caesarean delivery

- Psychological benefits of giving birth 'normally'. This is seen by some women as a nebulous entity, but is of great importance to many.
- Early attachment and bonding with the newborn, and the prompt establishment of breast feeding are best achieved after spontaneous delivery. Others dispute this, claiming the exhausted mother delivered after a prolonged labour or by caesarean section in labour

is less able to achieve this, compared to the woman after elective caesarean delivery.
- Neonatal respiratory distress. Provided the caesarean is scheduled for thirty-nine completed weeks gestation, this should be limited to transient tachypnea of the newborn with no longterm detriment.[12,13]
- Epidemiological studies have shown a modest increase in the risk of asthma, obesity and autoimmune disorders in children born by caesarean section.[14] These conditions are associated with alterations in the microbes that colonise the body, the microbiota, and has led to 'vaginal seeding' – the transfer of maternal vaginal fluid to the infant via a guaze wipe. This carries the potential risk of transferring pathogens, such as group B streptococcus, chlamydia and gonorrhoea.[15] Its role remains unclear.
- Longterm infant/childhood development may have subtle, as yet undelineated, advantages from labour and vaginal delivery.
- Maternal mortality and morbidity. A recent literature review suggests there is no significant difference in maternal mortality between vaginal delivery and elective caesarean section.[16]
- Cumulative maternal morbidity due to downstream complications of repeat caesarean delivery, including: uterine rupture, placenta praevia, placenta praevia accreta, and the need for hysterectomy. Placenta praevia accreta, in particular, is one of the most dangerous obstetric complications. These morbidities increase with successive caesarean sections, but only to a significant degree after three caesareans. [17,18]

Approach of health professionals to caesarean delivery by maternal choice

A number of surveys of the attitudes of obstetricians and midwives to caesarean section on maternal request have been published.[19-31] In summary these show the following:
- Obstetricians' willingness to perform caesarean section on maternal request: 15% - 81%. In three surveys male obstetricians were more willing than females to do the caesarean.
- Female obstetricians or obstetrical trainees who would request caesarean section themselves without medical indication: 9% - 31%. These figures rise considerably if the estimated fetal weight is high (>4000-4500g). The most common reasons for choosing elective caesarean delivery were fear of pelvic floor trauma and its sequelae,

and concern over neonatal damage.
- Midwives who would request caesarean on themselves: 4.5%. Midwives do not deal with the long-term sequelae of pelvic floor dysfunction.
- The number of pregnant women who would choose caesarean delivery if available: Nullipara 7.2% - 13%. Multipara 5% - 8.7%.

Economics of caesarean delivery

It is generally stated that caesarean delivery is more expensive than vaginal delivery; if all caesareans, those done electively without labour and those done as emergencies in labour, are lumped together this is quite true. But when elective caesareans without labour are costed separately the difference shrinks considerably.

In the United States, Bost compared the cost of nursing care and consumables in nulliparous women having an elective caesarean ($920) to those undertaking labour and planned vaginal delivery ($970).[32] Induction of labour and the need for caesarean section in labour accounted for the increased costs. If the woman had spontaneous labour and a vaginal delivery the cost fell to $780.[32] In the Term Breech Trial the total cost per mother/infant pair was $8402 for planned vaginal delivery and $7165 for planned caesarean.[33,34] We have analysed the cumulative costs of three deliveries, based on the type of labour (spontaneous, induced, none) and the method of delivery (spontaneous, assisted vaginal, elective caesarean, caesarean in labour) in the first pregnancy, in order to define the downstream obstetric costs.[35] The results are shown in the table:

First delivery	Cost of delivery 1	Cost of Dels 1&2	Cost of Dels 1,2&3
Type of labour	US$	US$	US$
- Spontaneous	2357	4781	6919
- Induced	2599	4982	7220
- No labour	2584	5306	7213
Method of delivery			
- Spontaneous	2124	4340	6425
- Assisted vaginal	2551	5230	7288
- Caesarean no labour	2584	5306	7213
- Caesarean in labour	3318	6319	9524

Over three pregnancies the cumulative costs of elective caesarean delivery without labour was 4.2% more than delivery after spontaneous labour (planned vaginal delivery). Compared to spontaneous delivery, elective caesarean section cost 12.3% more, assisted vaginal delivery 13.4% more and caesarean section in labour 48.2% more.[35]

The costs were applied per mother/infant pair and included all nursing costs in the antepartum, labour and delivery, postpartum and neonatal intensive care units, physician (obstetric, anaesthesia) costs, labour induction agents, consumables and cost of postpartum hysterectomy and tubal ligation.[35] This study emanated from within the Canadian publicly funded health service, and the physician fees for each type of labour or delivery were the same; therefore these figures may not apply to countries with health institutions run by for-profit corporations.

In essence, spontaneous labour and normal vaginal delivery is the most economic use of health resources, but if that outcome is not achieved, elective caesarean section is the next most economically favourable method of delivery.

If, indeed, the longterm maternal and perinatal morbidity is less with elective caesarean compared with planned vaginal birth, then the later costs of gynaecological surgery to correct prolapse and incontinence, plus the medical and litigation costs of the sequelae of fetal hypoxia and trauma (brachial plexus injury and cerebral palsy) should be added to the economic equation.[36] This would tip the overall economic balance in favour of elective caesarean delivery.

Ethics of caesarean delivery on maternal request

The ethical principles are straightforward, but the conclusions drawn from these principles after prolonged ethical discussion are often, in fact, inconclusive.[37] The physician is bound by the ethical code of beneficence (do good for the patient) and non-maleficence (do no harm to the patient). Along with these two guiding principles is a third and vital component – respect for the patient's autonomy. If the clinical factors are clear, the choice between good and harm is usually straightforward. The problem with caesarean delivery on maternal request is that the influencing factors are dictated by the often complex clinical profile of the individual patient: psychological factors, size of family desired, multiple risk factors for or against caesarean delivery.[38] Above all, what is the likelihood of this woman having a progressive labour and a normal spontaneous delivery- which is the only outcome with a safety profile for both mother and baby that comes close to that of planned elective caesarean section?

If, after this detailed appraisal, the obstetrcan concludes there is at least a balance between the potential benefit and harm of elective caesarean section, the decision to comply with her request is secure. The other overriding decision in this process is the fully informed consent of the woman. If the obstetrician feels that caesarean delivery carries potentially more harm than good, this must be outlined in detail with the patient. Being fully informed, if she still insists on caesarean delivery, most would acknowledge her autonomous right to that decision. However, the physician also has a right to autonomy and, if unwilling to do the caesarean, he/she can refuse but must refer her to another obstetrician.[39]

Physicians working within a publically funded health service also have a fiduciary duty not to squander finite health resources on un-indicated medical procedures. This was one of the reasons the ethics committee of the International Federation of Gynecologists and Obstetricians (FIGO) in 1998 stated, *'performing a cesarean delivery for non-medical reasons is ethically not justified.'* [40] They based this opinion, with a particular eye to developing countries, on the lack of proven benefit, additional longterm risks and the use of limited resources for obstetric care.[40] However, as detailed in the section above the economic argument against elective caesarean delivery is not valid – at least not in developed countries with a publically funded health service.

In terms of maternal morbidity, both in the first and subsequent pregnancies, and its cost to the health service, spontaneous vaginal delivery is the best choice. The serious perinatal/infant risks of intrapartum death, permanent brachial plexus injury and hypoxic ischaemic encephalopathy are also very low with spontaneous vaginal delivery, but virtually nil with elective caesarean section. In many ways this is the core of womens' choice caesarean delivery; they will always accept the higher risks of caesarean section for themselves, if it reduces the risk to their baby. It is difficult to provide them with hard reassuring facts on this point. For example, the risks of either intrapartum fetal death or permanent brachial plexus injury during labour and vaginal delivery is about 1 in 10,000.[41,42] This would exceed the threshold of perinatal risk acceptable to 22% of women in the previously quoted Australian study (see page 145); ie, if the risk of fetal death or permanent disability with labour and vaginal delivery was ≥ 1 in 10,000, they would request an elective caesarean section.[43]

The majority of the morbidity associated with planned vaginal delivery comes from those cases destined for assisted vaginal delivery with forceps or vacuum and, particularly with caesarean section in labour. Thus, if one could identify women most likely to have a progressive labour and spontaneous vaginal delivery, they would have the least maternal morbidity and come close to the lowest perinatal/infant risks of elective caesarean delivery. A small but emerging trend is the move to caesarean section on maternal request early in non-progressive labours.[44]

With elective caesarean section both the morbidity and economic costs rise considerably if the woman chooses to have more than three pregnancies. Thus, this component of the informed consent discussion is vital. The woman's decision must be informed by a detailed review of her psychological and clinical profile, leading to a reasoned benefit/harm calculation. However, the demographic profile of the obstetric population, at least in the developed world, has changed in a way that makes progressive labour and spontaneous vaginal delivery less likely (see chapter 14). Many of those who request elective caesarean delivery are older, educated women who have postponed pregnancy because of career development. We might therefore expect an increased demand for elective caesarean delivery from this group.

Finally, it does seem ironic that a woman has the right to refuse caesarean section when it is deemed advisable for her and her baby (see chapter 14), yet she may be refused the right to choose caesarean delivery for what she sees as the same reasons.

The reader is directed to a recent book on the subject, with balanced information aimed at both the lay and medical audience.[45]

REFERENCES

1. Humpstone OP. Cesarean section vs. spontaneous delivery. Am J Obstet Gynecol 1920;1:986-9.
2. Reynolds E. Primary operations for obstetrical debility. Surg Gynecol Obstet 1907;4:306-318.
3. Trolle D. The History of Caesarean Section. Copenhagen: C.A. Reitzel Booksellers; 1982. p39,56.
4. Claye A. Caesarean section – a lethal operation? J Obstet Gynaecol Br Commonw 1961;68:577-83.
5. Feldman GB, Freiman JA. Prophylactic cesarean section at term? N Engl J Med 1985;312:1264-7.
6. Hofberg K, Brockington I. Tokophobia: An unreasoning fear of childbirth: A series of 26 cases. Br J Psychiatry 2000;176:83-5.
7. Waldenstrom V, Hildingsson I, Ryding EL. Antenatal fear of childbirth and its association with subsequent caesarean section and experience of childbirth. BJOG 2006;113:638-46.

8. Hankins GD, Clark SM, Mann MB. Cesarean section on request at 39 weeks: Impact on shoulder dystocia, fetal trauma, neonatal encephalopathy, and intrauterine fetal demise. Semin Perinatol 2006;30:276-87.
9. Baskett TF, Allen VM, O'Connell CM, Allen AC. Fetal trauma in term pregnancy. Am J Obstet Gynecol 2007;197:499
10. Baskett TF, Allen VM, O'Connell CM, Allen AC. Predictors of respiratory depression at birth in the term infant. BJOG 2006;113:769-74.
11. Smith GC, Pell JP, Dobbie R. Caesarean section and risk of unexplained stillbirth in subsequent pregnancy. Lancet 2003;362:1779-84.
12. Alderdice F, McCall E, Bailie C et al. Admission to neonatal intensive care with respiratory morbidity following 'term' elective caesarean section. Irish Med J 2005;98:170-2.
13. Allen VM, Baskett TF, Allen AC et al. Type of labour in the first pregnancy and cumulative perinatal morbidity. J Obstet Gynaecol Can 2016;38:804-10.
14. Sevelsted A, Stokholm J, Bonnelykke K et al. Cesarean section and chronic immune disorders. Pediatrics 2015;135:e92-8.
15. Cunnington A, Sim K, Deierl A et al. "Vaginal seeding" of infants born by caesarean section. BMJ 2016;352:i227.
16. Vadnais M, Sachs B. Maternal mortality with cesarean delivery: a literature review. Semin Perinatol 2006;30:242-6.
17. Silver RM, Landon MB, Rouse DJ et al. Maternal morbidity associated with multiple repeat cesarean deliveries. Obstet Gynecol 2006;107: 1226-32.
18. Allen VM, Baskett TF, O'Connell CM. Type of labour in the first pregnancy and cumulative maternal morbidity. J Obstet Gynaecol Can 2015;35:688-95.
19. Al-Mufti R, McCarthy A, Fisk NM. Survey of obstetricians' personal preferences and discretionary practice. Eur J Obstet Gynaecol Reprod Biol 1997;73:1-4.
20. Dickson MJ, Willet M. Midwives would prefer a vaginal delivery (letter), BMJ 1999;176:254-5.
21. Wright JB, Wright AL, Simpson NA, Bryce FC. A survey of trainee obstetricians preferences for childbirth. Eur J Obstet Gynecol Reprod Biol 2001;97:23-5.
22. Groom KM, Paterson-Brown S, Fisk NM. Temporal and geographical variation in UK obstetricians' personal preference regarding mode of delivery. Eur J Obstet Gynecol Reprod Biol 2002;100:185-8.
23. Gonen R, Tamir A, Degani S. Obstetricians' opinions regarding patient choice in cesarean delivery. Obstet Gynecol 2002;99:577-80.
24. MacDonald C, Pinion SB, MacLeod UM. Scottish female obstetricians' views on elective caesarean section and personal choice for delivery. J Obstet Gynaecol 2002;22:586-9.
25. Hildingsson I, Radestad I, Rubertsson C, Waldenstrom U. Few women wish to be delivered by caesarean section. BJOG 2002;109:618-23.
26. Kwee A, Cohlen BJ, Kanhai HH et al. Caesarean section on request: a survey in The Netherlands. Eur J Obstet Gynecol Reprod Biol 2002;113:186-190.
27. Ghetti C, Chan BK, Guise JM. Physicians' responses to patient-requested

cesarean delivery. Birth 2004;31:280-4.
28. Pakenham S, Chamberlain SM, Smith GN. Women's views on elective primary caesarean section. J Obstet Gynaecol Can 2006;28:1089-94.
29. Farrell SA, Baskett TF, Farrell KD. The choice of elective caesarean delivery in obstetrics: a voluntary survey of Canadian health care professionals. Int J Urogynecol 2005;192:1475-7.
30. Pang MW, Lee TS, Leung AK et al. A longitudinal observational study of preference for elective caesarean section among nulliparous Hong Kong Chinese women. BJOG 2007;114:623-9.
31. Habiba M, Kaminski M, Fre MD et al. Caesarean section on request: a comparison of obstetricians attitudes in eight European countries. BJOG 2006;113:647-56.
32. Bost BW. Cesarean delivery on demand: what will it cost? Am J Obstet Gynecol 2003;188:1418-23.
33. Palencia R, Gafin A, Hannah ME et al. The costs of planned caesarean versus planned vaginal birth in the Term Breech Trial. CMAJ 2006;174:1109-13.
34. Henderson J, Petrou S. The economic case for planned caesarean section for breech presentation at term. CMAJ 2006;174:1118-9.
35. Allen VM, O'Connell CM, Baskett TF. Cumulative economic implications of initial method of delivery. Obstet Gynecol 2006;108:549-55.
36. Hale RW, Harer WB. Elective prophylactic cesarean delivery. ACOG Clinical Review. 2005;10:1, 15-16. American College of Obstetricians and Gynecologists, Washington DC.
37. Minkoff H, Powderly KR, Chervenak F, McCullough LB. Ethical dimensions of elective primary cesarean delivery. Obstet Gynecol 2004;103:387-92.
38. American College of Obstetricians and Gynecologists. Committee Opinion No.559. Cesarean delivery on maternal request. Obstet Gynecol 2013;121:904-7.
39. NICE Guideline. Caesarean section. London: Royal College of Obstetricians and Gynaecologists;2011.p96-103.
40. FIGO Committee Report. FIGO committee for the ethical aspects of human reproduction and women's health. Int J Obstet Gynecol 1999;64:317-32.
41. Mattatall FM, O'Connell CM, Baskett TF. A review of intrapartum fetal deaths. Am J Obstet Gynecol 2005;192:1475-7.
42. Chauhan SP, Rose CH, Gherman RB et al. Brachial plexus injury: a 23 year experience from a tertiary center. Am J Obstet Gynecol 2005;192:1795-1802.
43. Walker SP, McCarthy EA, Ugoni A et al. Cesarean delivery or vaginal birth: a survey of patient and clinical thresholds. Obstet Gynecol 2007;109:67-72.
44. Kalish RB, McCullough L, Gupta M et al. Intrapartum elective cesarean delivery: a previously unrecognized clinical entity. Obstet Gynecol 2004;103:1137-41.
45. Murphy M, Hull P. Choosing Cesarean: A Natural Birth Plan. Amherst, New York: Prometheus Books; 2012.

Chapter 16

Some caesarean 'firsts'

This final chapter will cover some of the known 'firsts' in the pantheon of caesarean birth. A number of these have been included in previous chapters:

First caesarean delivery by a lay person, 1500 (chapter 6);
First text on caesarean delivery, 1581 (chapter 8);
First authenticated caesarean section, 1610 (chapter 8);
First cattle horn caesarean, 1647 (chapter 5);
First suture of the uterine incision, 1769 (chapter 9);
First self-performed caesarean, 1769 (chapter 4);
First combined caesarean/vaginal twin delivery, 1822 (chapter 4);
First caesarean hysterectomy, 1869 (chapter 12).

First national caesarean deliveries

The first caesarean delivery in a living woman from individual countries can be hard to ascertain and verify. It is likely that many early and unsuccessful attempts went unrecorded. I have taken the following list from Trolle, with the operator in brackets – none of the mothers survived:[1]

- Germany (Jeremias Trautman, see chapter 8) 1610
- Sweden (Schützer) 1758
- Russia (Rhode) 1790
- Denmark (Schlegel, see chapter 15) 1813
- Norway (Backer) 1843
- Iceland (Hjaltolin) 1865

Other countries, for which there is more documentation, follow:

FRANCE

As noted in chapter 8, Rousset published a number of disputed cases occurring before 1581.[2] Ambroise Paré, although he advised against caesarean section, did acknowledge a successful case reported to him by reliable colleagues in 1542: *'I have, however, been assured that Master Vincent, a surgeon of Hericy near Fontainbleau, performed this operation with happy success.....As many persons of honour have related the fact to me and even affirmed that they saw him perform the operation and extract the infant, I cannot call their veracity into question.....'* [3] Mercurio and Guillemeau also noted caesarean deliveries in the latter part of the 1500s.[4,5] It therefore seems clear that some of the earliest attempts at caesarean section in living women took place in France in the mid/late 16th century.

BRITAIN

The first caesarean section in Great Britain was done on 29th June, 1737 by Robert Smith, a surgeon in Edinburgh. He was called to see an unfortunate woman, *'prodigiously deformed,'* with a distorted contracted pelvis that precluded all possibility of vaginal delivery. She had been in labour for six days and, after consultation with several colleagues, Smith did a caesarean section and delivered a large dead baby. The mother died eighteen hours later.[6] Apart from the successful case in 1738 by Mary Donally in Ireland (see chapter 6), it would be another fifty-six years before a woman survived caesarean delivery in the British Isles – ten other cases in the intervening years had all been fatal to the mother, although six infants were saved.[6]

The first English success came on 27th November 1793, when James Barlow (1767-1839), surgeon of Blackburn, Lancashire, operated on a patient with a traumatic pelvic deformity. The woman in question was forty year old Jane Foster, the mother of several children, who had been run over by a horse and cart sustaining severe pelvic fractures. She recovered sufficiently to get pregnant, but her obstructed labour was soon evident, and the severe nature of the pelvic contraction apparent to Barlow's examination. After consultation with a fellow surgeon the options were reviewed and they agreed that the only solution was caesarean section. However, the dangers of this so intimidated the other surgeon that *'.....he declined taking any part in it and he returned home.'* [7] Barlow found another surgeon to assist and proceeded to caesarean section. His task was made easier by Jane Foster's courage and forbearance: *'The poor woman scarcely complained during the operation, so great was her fortitude.'* [7] Not so his erstwhile assistant who *'.....was suddenly seized with a violent fit of syncope which wholly incapacitated him from attending to the steps of the operation and having no other professional person present I was obliged to be assisted by a female attendant.'* [7] The baby was in breech presentation and stillborn.

Mrs Foster's postoperative recovery was uneventful, she was allowed out of bed in two weeks and after another week had returned to her *'domestic duties.'* She had no further pregnancies and lived to be seventy-six years old.[7]

It is possible that the first caesarean section in England was done by one John Bullawnger, a yeoman of Buckden, Huntingdonshire.[8] He was charged in the Norfolk Assizes with causing the death of Agnes Redborne, *'spynster'*, by cutting open her abdomen and removing a baby on 17th June, 1573. He was accused of falsely claiming to be a surgeon – the outcome for the infant was not recorded, but the mother died ten days after the operation. Bullawnger was pardoned by the court on the basis of misadventure, because unqualified surgeons had practiced before the licensing of medical practitioners had come into effect.[8]

IRELAND

The first medically performed caesarean in Ireland was carried out in 1816 by Dr Charles Todd in Dublin; the baby survived but the mother died four days later. Two other cases were done in the North of Ireland with similar results. On 29th September 1829, a Dr McKibben did a caesarean section at the Belfast Lying-In Hospital, reputedly *'with great neatness, dexterity and calmness'*; however, the baby was stillborn and the mother died seventeen hours later.[9] In May 1849, Dr John Campbell was called to a *'wretched cabin'* near Dromara, County Down and confronted with a woman with osteomalacia and a contracted pelvis who had been in labour for two days. He did the caesarean under chloroform anaesthesia – the baby survived, but the mother died after eight days.[9,10]

The first caesarean delivery in Ireland with survival of both mother and baby was performed by Arthur Macan (1843-1908), Master of the Rotunda Hospital in Dublin. The patient was a twenty year old, single woman of small stature (3ft 8in). Using Listerian principles Macan did a classical caesarean section on 5th August, 1889; *'This was my first case, and I had never seen the operation performed.'*[11] He had, however, read Sanger's papers and followed that suture technique. The mother and baby did well.

SPAIN

The surgeon, Francisco Jaime Martinez did the first caesarean section on a live woman in Valencia in 1763.[12]

VENEZUELA

In 1820, in the region of Cumaná, Venezuela, the first recorded caesarean delivery of a living woman in Latin America was done by the Spanish surgeon, Alonso Ruiz Moreno. The mother died on the second postoperative day, but the child survived to the age of 80 years.[13]

UNITED STATES OF AMERICA

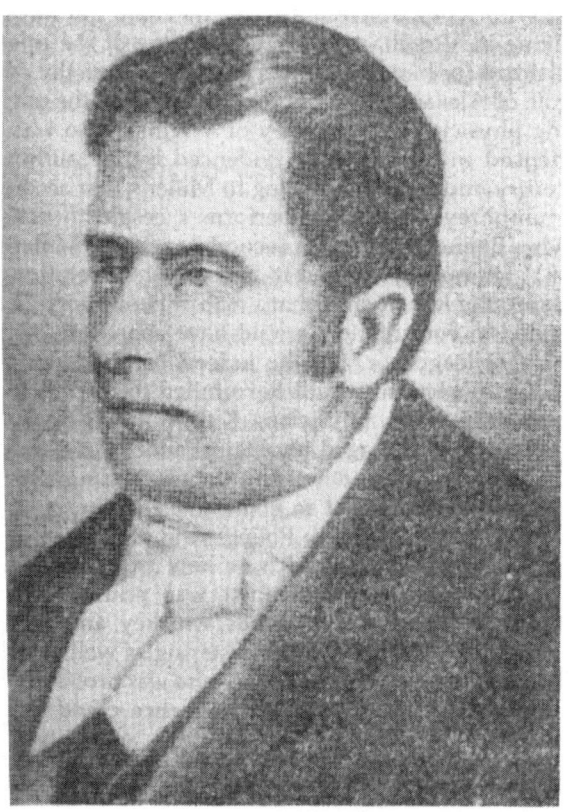

Figure 16.1
John Lambert Richmond (1785-1855)
In 1827, under epic circumstances, he performed the first caesarean section by a doctor in the United States

The first physician-performed caesarean with maternal survival was carried out by an unusual and engaging character: John Lambert Richmond (1785-1855). He was born in Chesterfield, Massachusetts into an impoverished family which moved frequently, seeking work and subsistence. Richmond received minimal formal schooling, but had access to books and was largely self educated. His family was very devout and in 1816 he was licensed as a Baptist minister. When the new Medical College of Ohio opened in 1820 Richmond enrolled as a student and as the assistant janitor. He graduated MD after 1½ years, moved to Newton, Ohio and doubled as the minister for the local Baptist church and doctor to the community.[14,15]

Many of the early caesarean deliveries in the United States, and most of the successful ones, were done by *'backwoods'* physicians. Indeed, Richmond published his case three years after the event in the Western Journal of the Medical and Physical Sciences, the motto of which was *E Sylvis Nuncius* or *'Messenger from the Backwoods.'* [15,16]

On the 22nd of April 1827, Richmond was called to a woman, *'Miss EC'*, who had been in labour for thirty hours. He rowed across the Little Miami River to her log cabin in the woods.[15,16]

'Two midwives had been called, but neither of them could give any account of the case, except that 'she had fits and the pains did no good."

The woman was having eclamptic convulsions, which he treated with laudanum and ether with reasonable effect, although she remained semi-comatose most of the time. He found the pelvic examination confusing, and it seems she had an anomalous lower genital tract causing soft tissue obstruction, that neither he or the labour could overcome. He was unable to get any professional advice or assistance on account of '….. *high water in the Little Miami and the darkness of the night.'* [16] It was, in fact, the proverbial *'dark and stormy night'*:

'Here I must take the liberty to digress from my subject, and relate the condition of the house, which was made of logs that were green, and put together not more than a week before. The crevices were not chinked, there was no chimney, nor chamber floor. The night was stormy and windy, insomuch, that the assistants had to hold blankets to keep the candles from being blown out.' [16]

After four hours Richmond '…..*was convinced that the patient must die, or the operation be performed…..I informed the patient and her friends, of the only means by which I could conceive of relief; this was at once consented to as affording some hopes of life.'*

He approached the operation:

'After doing all in my power for her preservation, and feeling myself entirely in the dark as to her situation, and finding that whatever was done, must be done soon, and feeling a deep and solemn sense of my responsibility, with only a case of common pocket instruments, about one o'clock at night, I commenced the caesarean section.' [16]

He made a lower midline incision in the abdomen, through the anterior wall of the uterus and the underlying placenta, but found it impossible to deliver the baby *'.....as it was uncommonly large, and the mother very fat, and having no assistance......'.*

The placenta became entirely detached and he still could not deliver the fetus. *'.....thinking the danger of the mother very great; and believing or supposing, that the child was dead from the detachment of the placenta; and considering, at all events, that a childless mother, was better than a motherless child, I determined to do all I could for preservation of the mother.'*

He therefore cut across the muscles of the back of the fetus, which permitted its delivery. He sutured the upper part of the abdominal incision, leaving the lower part open to drain: *'She now lay perfectly easy and went to sleep..... She commenced work in twenty-four days from the operation, and in the fifth week walked a mile and back the same day.'* [16]

From a man with no formal education and only eighteen months of theoretical medical training this article stands as a testament to logical decisive action under daunting circumstances, and to clear expressive writing – a case report for the ages.

In 1929, another challenger for the first medical caesarean section in the United States was put forward by Dr Joseph Miller.[17] The surgeon was stated to be Dr Jesse Bennet (1769-1842) of Virginia and the patient was his wife Elizabeth. On 14th January, 1794 Mrs Bennet, in her first pregnancy, had developed obstructed labour. Attempted forceps delivery was unsuccessful and she asked for caesarean section rather than craniotomy. Jesse Bennet performed the caesarean and delivered his daughter, he also removed the ovaries to avoid a repeat performance; both mother and daughter survived. Miller published another report in 1938, after an obstetric text was *'found in the attic,'* with a few cryptic notes said to be by the hand of Bennet: *'14 Jan 1794 JB on EB. Up 9 Feb Walked 15 Feb Cured on 1 March.'* [18] The text, an English translation of Baudelocque, was an 1801 edition – seven years after the operation. The whole episode has since been subjected to detailed scrutiny by Dr Arthur King, an obstetrician from Cincinnati, who cast considerable doubt on the veracity of the above event.[19] It seems the whole episode rests on the story told by Jesse Bennet's sister-in-law, Mrs Nancy Hawkins, as recounted to a Dr Aquilla Knight some fifty-three years after the fact. He, in turn, only wrote of this encounter after another forty-five years, in 1892.[20] Knight, who died in 1897, told the story to a youthful Joseph Miller, who did not publish his account until 1929.[17]

King could find no documented evidence that the caesarean operation had been performed, and between Miller's and another account of Bennet's life [21] he found many discrepancies. There was no record of Bennet having studied medicine in Philadelphia as Miller stated; he was described more as a general storekeeper who sold medications and carried out bleeding and blistering on the side.[21] As such he may have been known to the locals as 'Doc'. He kept detailed notes of his inventory, sales, bleeding and blistering – but no mention of any surgical procedures.[21] Thus, the caesarean event rests entirely on hearsay from Bennet's sister-in-law, given fifty-three years after the event. It is possible that the Bennet caesarean saga is true, but the lack of supporting evidence, and the numerous discrepancies unearthed by King, make it unlikely.[19]

COLUMBIA

In the Medellin region of Columbia in 1844, Dr Jose Ignacio Quevedo performed the first caesarean section with survival of both mother and child.[13]

AUSTRALIA

The first caesarean section in Australia came as a surprise to the surgeon, Thomas Hillas (1827-1892), at the Ballarat District Hospital.[22,23] The patient, an impoverished, single, twenty-four year old immigrant from Cork in Ireland, had been admitted to the Ballarat Benevolent Asylum thinking herself to be pregnant. Seven months later the doctors decided she was not pregnant but had a large ovarian cyst; she was therefore transferred to the District Hospital.[22] At laparotomy on 13th June 1872 it turned out that both the patient and the doctors were correct; she had a large ovarian cyst (containing 11 litres of fluid) and a term pregnant uterus. The ovarian cyst was easily removed and, because of an inadvertent incision in the uterine wall during entry to the abdomen, Hillas extended that incision and performed a classical caesarean section. He used silver wire sutures to close the uterine incision and the mother's recovery was uncomplicated. The baby was delivered alive and *'of about eight month's development'* – but its longterm outcome was not recorded.[22]

John Cooke (1850-1921), who had trained in London and came to Australia as a ships surgeon in 1873, did the first planned caesarean section at the Alfred Hospital in Melbourne.[22,23] The patient was a forty-three year old mother of ten, in labour for eighteen hours with a cancerous growth occluding the vagina. *'The only chance of saving the woman's and child's life was the operation resorted to.'*[22] On 20th March, 1885 Cooke did a classical caesarean section and delivered a 7lb baby girl who was well, but died of gastroenteritis after discharge from hospital. The mother survived.

The first planned Porro caesarean hysterectomy was performed by another English trained surgeon, Walter Balls-Headley (1842-1918), who came to Australia because of chronic lung disease and the damp English climate. At the Women's Hospital, Melbourne on 14th October, 1886 he carried out the procedure with success on a rachitic dwarf. The mother's recovery was complete within two months. The baby girl did well, but had the misfortune to be given the Christian names, Porrina Balls-Headley.[22]

MEXICO

The rarity of caesarean delivery is shown by the fact there were only three documented cases between 1877 and 1897. The first took place in Monterey in September 1877 and was carried out by consulting surgeons JB and JH Mears, called in by the local physician. The indication was obstructed labour due to exostosis of the sacrum and failed craniotomy. The mother survived.[12,24]

The first Porro caesarean hysterectomy was done on 12th March, 1884 by Juan Maria Rodriguez, Professor of Clinical Obstetrics at the National School of Medicine in Mexico City. The patient was a rachitic dwarf, in labour and with an impassable contracted pelvis. The operation was carefully planned by Rodriguez, with a total of thirteen assistants to cover each aspect of perioperative care – including the *'provision of warm clothes.'* The baby girl cried immediately at birth, and was baptised *'Nonnato Porro Rodriguez.'* The mother died the following day.[12,24] The next caesarean on a live woman was in Merida, Yucatan in 1897 by Eudaldo Ferraez – the baby was stillborn and the mother died shortly thereafter.

MALTA

The first caesarean on a live woman, yet another rachitic dwarf, was performed by the Professor of Midwifery at the University of Malta, GB Schembri, on 28th May 1891, at the Central Hospital, Floriana. The patient was in labour and the cervix fully dilated on a *'markedly restricted rachitic pelvis.'*[25] After consultation with three other physicians Professor Schembri did a classical caesarean section under chloroform anaesthesia. Both mother and infant survived.

CUBA

In 1900, Enrique Fortun Andre (1872-1947), the Professor of Pathological Surgery at the University of Havana, did the first successful caesarean section with survival of both mother and child. In the same year, LeRoy Cassa, carried out the first Porro operation.[26]

SINGAPORE

In 1907 the maternity unit at The Kandang Kerbau Hospital had no operating theatre, so the first patient to have a caesarean section (for transverse lie) had to be transferred to the General Hospital.[27]

MALAWI

The Scottish surgeon, H.D. Cronyn, performed the first caesarean section, under spinal anaesthesia, in Zomba in 1936.[28]

First caesarean by a cross dresser

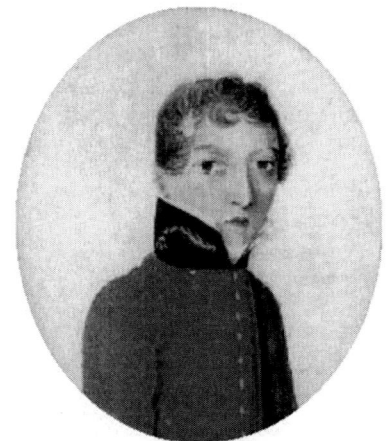

Figure 16.2
James Barry MD, (1789-1865)
Performed the first successful caesarean section in South Africa in 1826

On 25th July 1826, James Barry MD, (1789-1865) assistant surgeon in the British Army at Cape Town, South Africa, performed the first caesarean section in that colony, with survival of both mother and child. Barry had been posted to Cape Town in 1816 and gained a high reputation as a surgeon with obstetrical experience. The patient, Wilhelmina Munnik came from an old colonial family and her husband was a wealthy snuff manufacturer. Mrs Munnik was in labour with her first pregnancy; the details are not documented but she was in great pain and her life deemed to be in danger. James Barry was called and quickly made a decision that delivery should be by caesarean section, which he carried out on the kitchen table. Mother and child recovered uneventfully. Barry was offered a handsome fee by the grateful husband, but declined and asked only that the child be named after him. Thus, James Barry Munnik was baptised on 20th August, 1826. The Munnik family continued to name the firstborn male James Barry. A grandson, James Barry Munnik Hertzog, was prime minister of South Africa from 1924 to 1939.[29]

Barry was of small stature, smooth-faced, with a high pitched voice and these feminine qualities were only confirmed after '*his*' death in 1865. Barry died in London of dysentery and it was the Irish maid, Sophia Bishop, who laid out his body and declared that the corpse was that of '*a perfect female.*' Barry was buried in Kensal Green Cemetery, London without further examination.

James Barry had managed a fifty-two year career as an army surgeon without his secret being detected. After Cape Town he served in Mauritius, Jamaica, Malta, Corfu and finally as Inspector-General of Hospitals for Upper and Lower Canada – based in Montreal. From Canada he retired back to London on half pay.[30] How he came to be in Cape Town as a military surgeon has recently been clarified by Michael du Preez, a retired urologist from that city.[31] The Barrys were from Cork in Ireland. Mary Ann Barry married Jeremiah Bulkley and her second child, a daughter, was born in 1789. Bad investment and debts incurred by the oldest son, put Jeremiah in debtors prison in 1804 and left Mary Ann Bulkley and her daughter Margaret Ann destitute. They moved to London and found help from Mary Ann's brother, James Barry – an artist of good reputation. He also had a number of influential and liberal minded friends, including a doctor and a Venezuelan revolutionary general. They ensured that Margaret Ann got a sound education and, when James Barry died in 1806, mother and daughter had sufficient funds to remain in London. The doctor and the general devised a plan for Margaret Ann Bulkley to study medicine and ultimately go to Venezuela as a revolutionary army doctor. The problem was that females were not admitted to study medicine at that time. Thus, in November 1809 the young Margaret Ann Bulkley dressed as a young man, '*James Barry,*' and took the boat from London with his '*aunt*', Mary Ann Bulkley, to Leith in Scotland and enrolled at Edinburgh's medical school.[31] This was sixty years before Sophie Jex-Blake and her companions became the first female medical students in Britain.[32] James Barry qualified MD from Edinburgh University in 1812 – defending his thesis on femoral hernia in Latin. This was followed by six month as a surgeon's pupil at St Thomas' Hospital in London. By this time the Venezuelan general was dead so that avenue of employment was closed. Thus, James Barry, who had managed to sustain his male persona for three years, joined the British Army as a hospital assistant.[31] A recent book on this fascinating tale is recommended.[33]

First caesarean for placenta praevia

Lawson Tait (1845-1899), Professor of Gynaecology at Queen's College, Birmingham, was one of the most audacious, opinionated and successful gynaecological surgeons of his era – characteristics that were bound to make him enemies. Upon reviewing the morbidity and mortality associated with vaginal accouchement forcé and placenta praevia in 1890 he wrote:

'If I had to deal with a case of placenta praevia from the beginning of labour, and could carry out what I believe would be the ideal surgical treatmen, of this condition, I should amputate the pregnant uterus. I should thereby save the child with certainty. I should relieve the mother with perfect safety from death by haemorrhage; and by removing all the tissues in which large suppurating sinuses were present, I believe I should relieve her with almost equal certainty from the secondary risks.' [34]

Predictably, his suggestion was met with almost universal opposition, particularly in Britain. Tait did not have an opportunity to put his theory into practice until 1898, with survival of mother and baby.[35]

In the meantime the *'backwoods'* surgeons of the United States forged ahead. Although the exact date and details are unknown, it seems the first caesarean for placenta praevia was carried out by Drs Hypes and Hulbert of St Louis. The result was fatal, as it was done as a last resort, *'under the most unfavourable circumstances,'* and was never documented in detail.[36] Dr J Sligh of Granite City, Montana did record his caesarean section, done on 9th November, 1891. The patient, a para 4, presented with labour pains and bleeding off and on for one week at *'about seven months'* gestation. Sligh found a rigid, unyielding cervix which he felt was probably cancerous. All attempts at achieving vaginal delivery failed, and the baby presented as a transverse lie with a complete placenta praevia. At this point he advised caesarean delivery, but offered only *'.....the slightest hope for recovery because of the patient's condition, her surroundings (being in a boarding house), and a suspicion, approaching a diagnosis, that the exceedingly resistant condition of the neck was due to carcinoma.'* [37] He did a classical caesarean section, but his prognosis was correct and the mother died within twelvd hours. He concluded his report with the opinion that had he moved to caesarean sooner, *'.....it is probable that the patient's chances for life would have been better.'* [37]

Augustus Charles Bernays, Professor of Obstetrics at St Louis, Missouri had read and been impressed by the 1892 paper of Hutson Ford, which laid out the theoretical basis for treating complete placenta praevia with caesarean section.[38] He had this in mind when he was called on 19th November, 1893 to a woman at thirty-six weeks gestation who had just had her second haemorrhage in twelve hours – despite rest and vaginal temponade.[36]

'Found the patient excited and frightened by the unexpected haemorrhage, sitting in a chair and a large bundle of clothes under her saturated with blood.....The os was closed but the finger could be introduced and the placenta felt, as well as the blood streaming from the uterus.'

All six physicians present agreed that caesarean section '*.....was the best thing for the mother and child under the existing circumstances.*' The mother was a healthy forty-two year old with four children, and the house was *'newly –built'* so they prepared a room for the operation. Using chloroform and Lister's principles, Professor Bernays did a classical section without complication. The baby was born in good condition but died within twelve hours, probably from a congenital heart defect. The mother recovered without incident.[36]

REFERENCES

1. Trolle D. The History of Caesarean Section. Copenhagen: C.A. Reitzell Booksellers;1982.
2. Rousset F. Traitte Nouveau de L'Hysterotomotokie ou Enfantement Caesarien. Paris: Denys du Val;1581.
3. Johnston TH. English Translation of the Works of Ambroise Parey. London: T. Cotes and R. Young;1634.
4. Mercurio S. La Commare O Riccoglitrice. Venice: Ciotti;1596.
5. Guillemeau J. L'Heureux Accouchement des Femmes. Paris: Abraham Picord;1598. (Translated into English in 1612 by Thomas Hatfield as The Happy Delivery of Women. London;1612).
6. Young JH. Caesarean Section: The History and Development of the Operation from Earliest Times. London: HK Lewis & Co Ltd;1944.p36-7.
7. Naqui NH. James Barlow (1767-1839): operator of the first successful caesarean section in England. BJOG 1985;92:468-72.
8. Pugh RB. An early case of caesarean section in England. J Obstet Gynaecol Br Emp 1949;56:872-4.
9. Gibson GB. Caesarean birth. Ulster Med J 1962;31:57-63.
10. O'Sullivan JF. Caesarean birth. Ulster Med J 1990;59:1-10.
11. Macan AV. A case of successful caesarean section. Trans Roy Acad Med Ireland 1890;8:307-12.
12. Uribe-Elias R. The cesarean operation in Mexico. In: Viesca T (ed). Historia de Medicina en Mexico. Universidad Nacional Autonoma de Mexico: Mexico;p299-311.

13. Sanchez TF. The first cesarean section in Columbia. In: Sanchez TF. History of Gynaecology and Obstetrics in Columbia. Editorial La Portada,1993.
14. Robinson V. The Story of Medicine. New York: Tudor Publishing Co;1931. p469-70.
15. King AG. America's first cesarean section. Obstet Gynecol 1971;37:797-802.
16. Richmond JL. History of a successful case of Casarean Operation. Western J Med Phys Sci 1830;3:485-9.
17. Miller JL. Dr Jesse Bennet (1769-1842) pioneer surgeon, and Dr Aquilla Leighton Knight (1823-1896) humanist. Virginia Med Monthly 1929;55:711-4.
18. Miller JL. Caesarean section in Virginia in the pre-aseptic era, 1794-1879. Am Med Hist 1938;10:23-35.
19. King AG. The legend of Jesse Bennet's 1894 caesarean section. Bull Hist Med 1976;50:242-50.
20. Knight AL. The life and times of Jesse Bennet MD. Southern Hist Mag 1892;2:1-13.
21. Poling D. Jesse Bennet, pioneer physician and surgeon. West Virginia Hist 1951;12:87-128.
22. Forster FMC. Caesarean section and its early Australian history. Med J Aust 1970;2:33-8.
23. Proust AJ. A Companion of the History of Medicine in Australia 1788-1939. Melbourne: A.J. Proust;2003.p85.
24. Castelazo AL. History of Gynecology and Obstetrics in Mexico. Monograph: Mexican Federation of Obstetrics and Gynecology;1970.
25. Savona-Ventura C. Caesarean section in the Maltese Islands. Med Hist 1993;37:37-55.
26. Lugones BM. Cesarean section in history. Rev Cubana Obstet Ginecol 2001;27:53-6.
27. Tan KH (ed). The History of Obstetrics and Gynaecology in Singapore. Singapore: Armour Publishing;2003.p302-4.
28. King MS, King E. The Story of Medicine and Disease in Malawi. London: Daunt Books;1992.p165.
29. Holmes R. Scanty Particulars: The Scandalous Life and Astonishing Secret of Queen Victoria's Most Eminent Military Doctor. New York: Random House;2002.p152-61.
30. Cronin RPF. The strange case of Dr James Barry. Ann R Coll Phys Surg Can 2001;34:444-7.
31. Du Preez HM. Dr James Barry: The early years revealed. S Afr Med J 2008;98:52-8.
32. Crowther MA, Dupree MW. Medical Lives in the Age of Surgical Revolution. Cambridge: Cambridge University Press;2007:p8.
33. Du Preez HM, Dronfield J. Dr James Barry: A Woman Ahead of Her Time. London: OneWorld Publication;2016.
34. Tait L. The surgical treatment of impacted labour. BMJ 1890;1:657-9.

35. Tait L. On the treatment of 'unavoidable haemorrhage' by removal of the uterus. Lancet 1899;1:364-5.
36. Bernays AC. The first successful case of caesarean section in placenta praevia, and remarks on the method of operation. JAMA 1894;22:687-8.
37. Sligh JM. Placenta previa, cesarean section, absolute indication. Am J Obstet Dis Woman Child 1892;25:221-3.
38. Ford WH. Cesarean section and complete placenta previa. Am Gynecol J 1892;2:525-7.

Index

Abortion, and contracted pelvis 61
Aburel, Eugen 134
Accouchement forcé 75
Aesculapius 1-2
Aitken, John 83
Albiruni 44
Albucasis 44
Anaesthesia
   balanced 133
   epidural 135,146,160
   local 133-4
   spinal 134-5
Antibiotic prophylaxis 140
Anti-caesarean school 65-6
Antisepsis 67,72-5,84,90,123
Apollo 1-2, 66
Aquinas, Thomas 42
Aranzi, Guilo (Arantius) 59-61
Asepsis 67,72-3
Astruc, Jean 18
Aurelia 6
Auto-caesarean section 23

Bacchus 1-2
Balls-Headingly, Walter 175-6
Baptism 16-20,41-3
Bard, Samuel 56, 61, 147
Barlow, James 87, 170-1
Barry, James 177-8
Baudelocque, Jean-Louis 17, 63, 66, 83-4, 86-7, 94, 174
Baudelocque, Louis-August 98
Bauhin, Gaspard 34,49
Beck, Alfred 115
Bennett, Jesse 174-5
Bernard of Gordon 13
Bernays, Charles 179-80
Bier, August 134
Bloodletting 83,128
Blood transfusion 139
Blundell, James 120, 128, 139, 152-3
Brachial plexus injury 8,165
Breech and caesarean delivery 144-5
Bruce, Marjory 3
Buddha 2
Bullawnger, John 171

Bullekerk (Bull Church) 30
Bupivicaine 135
Burton, John 64

Caesar, Augustus 8
Caesar, Julius 6
Caesarean hysterectomy 67, 74, 112-3,119-26,152,175-6
Caesarean section and
   cardio-pulmonary resuscitation 20
   and Catholic church 16-19, 41-4,64,70
   and Hinduism 45
   and informed consent 82,148, 152-3,165-6
   and inheritance law 16,19-20
   and Islam 44-5
   and Judaism 40-1
   and litigation 148,164
   and newborn kidnapping 29
   cattle-horn 29-31
   classical 89-91,98,112,113, 116, 125, 141,175
   extraperitoneal 97-101,110
   indications 145
   lower segment 107-117,141
   perimortem 20-1
   postoperative care 94-5
   prophylactic 160
   rates 148-51
   ten-group classification 145-6
   vaginal 104-5
Cameron, Murdoch 91-3
Cangiamila, Francesco 43
Castro, Rodrigo de 15
Cazeaux, Paulin 58,70
Celsus 7,12
Chapman, Edmund 56
Charpentier, A 18
Chauliac, Guy de 13-14,16
Chiron 1
Chloroform 119,121,130-1,171
Cocaine 133-4
Coffin birth 13
Cohnheim, Isidor 85
Compelled caesarean delivery 153-4

Coronis 1
Craigin, Edwin 76,151
Craniotomy 44,62,64,67,70-1,74,94
Cyr, Ronald 49,150-1

Davey, Humphrey 131
DeLee, Joseph 115-6,134
Denman, Thomas 56,65,152
Dewees, William 56,69, 98-9, 128
Dionis, Pierre 15-17,55,60
Dipthong 9
Donally, Mary 36,170
Dubois, Antoine 44
Duhrssen, Alfred 104-5
Dystocia 144-7

Eclampsia 75-6,173
Economics of method of delivery 163-5
Embryotomy 62-4,70,74
Ergometrine 140
Ergot 87,140
Essen-Moller, Elis 75-6
Ether anaesthesia 122,130-2,173
Ethics and method of delivery 164-6
Extrauterine pregnancy 35,47

Felkin, Robert 36-9
Ferdowsi, Hakim 3,44
Fetal entrapment 85-6
Fetal indications for caesarean delivery 143-4,161
Forceps
   high 72,144
   mid 144,165
Foster, Jane 170-1
Frank, Fritz 102,113

Garriques, Henry 91
Giffard, William 56
Glasgow Maternity Hospital 91-3

Index

Guillemeau, Jacques 9,50,54,170

Halstead, William 73,134
Hammurabi 11-12
Harris, Robert 31-2,51, 68-70,75,82,88-9
Harvey, William 13
Henry VIII 3-4
Heparin 141
Heretic baptism 42
Hillas, Thomas 175
Hippocrates 12,40,129
Holinshed, Raphael 4
Holland, Eardley 114-5
Hôtel Dieu 42
Hull, John 66-7
Humpstone, Paul 159

Incision
  abdominal 84-5,98,101,113
  uterine 85-6,87-93,101,112 115,142
Induction of labour 61,70,146
Inheritance law 16,19-20
International Federation of Gynecologists and Obstetricians (FIGO) 165
Isidore of Seville 7

Jeffcoate, Norman 151-2
Johnson, Robert 107
Kaiserschnitt 8
Kaiser Wilhelm II 8
Kayser, Carl 57
Kehrer, Adolf 87,91,94,104,107,110-3
Kelly, Howard 56
Kerr, Munro 74-5,103-4,116-7,132
King Blearie 3
Klilovich, Stanislav 131
Koch, Robert 72
Koller, Carl 133
Kreis, Oscar 134

La Motte, Guillaume 62-3
Latzko, Wilhelm 100-1
Laudanum 122,129,173

Lauverjat, Théodore-Etienne 64,76

Lebas, Jean 87
Lee, Robert 56
Leopold, Christian 91
Lex caesarea 9,11,16
Lex regia 8,11,13
Lister, Joseph 72-3,90-1
Lucina 4,66

Macan, Arthur 171
Macauley, George 61
Maha, Maya 2
Malacosteon 58
Marchant, Jacques 50
Marshall, McIntosh 103,116,133-5
Martin, Eduard 8
Maternal demographics 146-8
Maternal mortality 27,31,57,67 69,72,74-5,88,105,122,126,133 136-8,143,162
Maternal threshold for clinical risk 148,165
Mauriceau, Francois 20,55
Maygrier, Jacques-Pierre 73,85
Mendelson's syndrome 133
Mercurio, Scipio 51-4,60-1,94,170
Misgav Ladach caesarean technique 143
Misoprostol 140
Mollites ossium 58
Moore, James 129
Munnik, Wilhelmina 177-8

Napoleon 44
Neonatal respiratory distress 162
Neufer, Elizabeth 35
Neufer, Jakob 34-5,47
Newborn kidnapping 29
Nitrous oxide 122,131-2
Noble, Charles 75
Nonnatus, Raymond 9
Numa Pompilius 8,11,13

Obstetrical Society of London 56-7
O'Neal, Alice 36
Opium 94,123,129
Osiander, Friedrich 82,107-9
Osteomalacia 58,171

Ould, Fielding 55
Oxytocin 140

Paré, Ambroise 49-50,54,169-70
Pasteur, Louis 72
Pelvis
  contracted 58-61,74,76,83,97, 109,170
  and craniotomy 62,70-1
  and induced abortion 61
  and induction of labour 61,70
  Naegele's 58
  Robert's 58
  and symphysiotomy 62
Perinatal mortality 58,62,69,72,148 164-5
Peritoneal closure 142
Peritoneal exclusion techniques 102-3
Peritonitis 24,103-4,113-4,125
Placenta and caesarean section 86,103 142
Placenta praevia 75,104,126,144, 179-80
Playfair, William 71-2,83,86,130
Pliny, the Elder 6-7
Polin, Frank 88
Porro, Edoardo 120-3
Portal, Paul 42
Portes operation 104
Posthumous caesarean delivery 154
Postpartum ambulation 140-1
Postpartum haemorrhage 86-7,119,140
Priestley, Joseph 131
Prontosil 140
Prostaglandins 140
Pubiotomy 62

Radford, Thomas 67,69-71,82, 85-6,130
Raynaud, Theophilus 54
Richmond, John 172-4
Rickets 58-61,83,91,109
Rigby, Edward 57
Ritgen, August von 97-8

Index

Robert II, King of Scotland 3
Robson, Michael 145,150
Rodenstein, Charles 88
Rodriquez, Juan 176
Roonhuyse, Hendrick von 20,64
Rosslin, Euharius 14
Rostam 3
Rotunda Hospital Dublin 76-7,171
Roudabeth 3
Rousset, Francois 9,32,34,47-51,55 85,87,94
Routh, Amand 74-5,104

Sacombe, Jean-Francois 65-6
Samhita 12,45
Sanger, Max 87,89-94,102,112,125
Schwarz, Ignaz 18019
Sebezius, Melchoir 49
Selheim, Hugo 102
Semele 2
Sennert, Daniel 54
Sepsis and caesarean delivery 73-4,140
Serterner, Friedrich 129
Seymour, Jane 3
Shahnameh (Book of Kings) 3
Shakespeare, William 4
Sharp, Jane 15
Sigurdsson, Jon 16
Simmons, William 66-7
Simpson, James 130-1
Simulation training 12
Skene, Alexander 100
Smellie, William 62,64
Smith, Robert 170
Smith, Tyler 70-1
Soranus 12
Spencer, Herbert 76-7,131
Spiegelberg, Otto von 83,86,94
Spongia somnifera 129
Sterilisation 125,152-3
Stillbirth 69,161,165
Stoeckel, Walter 134
Storer, Horatio 119-20,132
Supine hypotension syndrome 135
Sushruta 12

Suture material 87-8,90-1,113,142
Symphysiotomy 62,65
Tait, Lawson 179
Thiopental 132-3
Thomas, Theodore Gaillard 99-100
Thromboprophylaxis 140-1
Tocophobia 161
Trautmann, Jeremias 54
Tubal ligation and caesarean section 153
Tuohy, Edward 135
Twins and caesarean delivery 145

Uganda 37
Uterine incision
 closure 87,94,111-12,116,142
 type 112,115,141,143
Uterine massage 86-7
Uterine rupture 107-8,115-6,126,146
Uterine suture 67,73,87-91
Utero-abdominal fistula 102

Vacuum assisted delivery 144
Vaginal birth after caesarean (VBAC) 23,28,31,35,41,51,141,151-2
Vaginal caesarean section 104-5
Vaginal 'seeding' 162
Velpeau, Louis 64,128
Venice, Senate of 18
Ventricular fibrillation 132
Volpe, Isabella Della 19
Volsungs 3

Warfarin 141
Williams, John Whitridge 75,77,153
Willoughby, Percival 54-5,60
Wood, Alexander 129
World Health Organization(WHO) 149-51
Zaandam 29
Zal 3
Zeus 2